ONLY SKIN DEEP?

For one of my
best friends —
Kathleen, you have
been a source of
strength and comfort,
a person to laugh with,
cry with, grow with, and
enjoy this thing called
friendship with — Thank you.

Love
Danielle

ONLY SKIN DEEP?

✦

An Essential Guide to Effective Skin Cancer Programs and Resources

By *Danielle M. White*

Foreword by Clay J. Cockerell, M.D.

Afterword by Melissa Burns

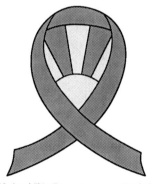

National Skin Cancer Awareness Symbol

iUniverse, Inc.
New York Lincoln Shanghai

ONLY SKIN DEEP?
An Essential Guide to Effective Skin Cancer Programs and Resources

iUniverse books may be ordered through booksellers or by contacting:

iUniverse
2021 Pine Lake Road, Suite 100
Lincoln, NE 68512
www.iuniverse.com
1-800-Authors (1-800-288-4677)

First Edition

ISBN: 978-0-595-43273-8 (pbk)
ISBN: 978-0-595-87613-6 (ebk)

Printed in the United States of America

For Natalie

Contents

Acknowledgements

My sincerest appreciation to everyone who extended time, talents, efforts, energy, and resources, whether it be monetarily or in-kind, on behalf of The Cancer Crusaders Organization since we officially incorporated in January 2004, and, specifically, toward the completion of this book.

Thank you to the faculty and staff at Utah Valley State College, especially: Dr. Christa Albrecht-Crane, Phil Clegg, and Dr. Mark Jeffreys who served on my Senior Thesis board and helped, believe it or not, create a sound foundation for the beginning of this book. Thank you, Christa (the self-proclaimed "MLA Nazi") for your abundant talent and sheer brilliance, and for pushing me to excel beyond my known capacities. You are, perhaps, the smartest person I have ever known; a true genius. Thank you, also, to the wonderful crew in the UVSC College Marketing Department, particularly Melynda Thorpe-Burt for your enthusiastic support and for helping us spread the word about the National Skin Cancer Awareness Symbol© via the alumni magazines. To Dr. Janice Gygi and Derek Hall (even though, Derek has since moved on to "greener pastures") for making it possible for us to attend the 2005 Gold Triangle Awards ceremony in Chicago and, as such, see a dream of a universally accepted Skin Cancer Awareness ribbon symbol be realized. Thanks to Dr. Sam Rushforth and Dr. Ruhul Kuddus in the UVSC Science and Health Department, and to my ever-kind, generous, and insightful college mentor Nancy Plagge for believing that I could succeed at any endeavor I attempted. Many thanks to the UVSC School of Business for the donation of office space in the student incubators to help us function. (Shauna Theobald—you are missed). And to my cubicle neighbors—Bart, David, John, and Ryan—for putting up with my pushing samples of Blue Lizard Australian Sunscreen and skin cancer information literature upon you, and for letting me drape orange-and-yellow Skin Cancer Awareness ribbons over every inch of our office space.

Thank you to the media—Jeanette at Bennett Communications, Jeff at the *Deseret News*, Christy at the *Salt Lake Tribune*, Chad, Christina, and Kim at the Grapevine Talk Radio Network, Tiffany from Succeeding Gracefully, Curt and Zach from the Paradigm, along with *The Daily Universe* at Brigham Young University, and *SHAPE* Magazine. Thank you for helping us to introduce the new national Skin Cancer Awareness ribbon symbol to the masses. A great deal of gratitude goes to our partners at Grapevine Radio for the opportunity of launching the award-winning *"Conversations with Cancer"* show and thus providing a medium by which we could launch the "ONLY SKIN DEEP?"® Peer Educator's Training and Certification Program.

Thank you to our sponsors past and present: Bennett Communications, Central Utah Clinic, Corporate Alliance, Crowell Advertising, Crown Laboratories and Del-Ray Dermatologicals (the makers of Blue Lizard Australian Sunscreen), GT Advantage, Grapevine Talk Radio Network, Healthy Wealthy Wow, Hudson Incorporated, Local Appeal, NeoStrata, Sun Safety Alliance, and Utah Valley State College. We are deeply grateful to Jeff Bedard and Keisha Bratton at Del-Ray Dermatologicals for their genuine commitment to skin cancer efforts and for their wonderful friendship. If only every business in America were run after the manner in which Del-Ray is—by individuals who truly care about serving their communities and do so with great zeal, in addition to providing high quality, trusted products. I bleed "Blue [Lizard]" for you.

Thank you to my pageant girls and to my students—Brittany and Carly for the support; Erika for [reluctantly] foregoing your tanning habit (and for the great memories filled with lots of laughter); Kaylan, for being a shining example to other contestants about the importance of protecting your skin; Maile, for the remarkable work you are doing at Southern Utah University and the surrounding community. Thank you for representing The Cancer Crusaders Organization, and the cause, so well; Hoku, Nani, and Sunshine, if it weren't for the three of you the peer education program would never have lifted from the ground.

To our respected and admired colleagues at the American Academy of Dermatology; it is a privilege to work with each of you. Thank you, especially, to Connie Tegeler, Jennifer Allyn, Lisa Doty, and Laura Edwards. We applaud and salute the AAD for setting the standard of excellence in the dermatology field and acknowledge the AAD as the leading experts for accurate, updated information on dermatologic health.

Thank you to our fellow skin cancer crusaders at the Coalition, the National Council on Skin Cancer Prevention, the Sun Safety Alliance, "ONE VOICE" for Melanoma, the Environmental Protection Agency, and the Women's Dermatologic Society, and to each of the active melanoma foundations throughout the United States. My regards to Beverly Berkin (SSA); Robin Lawrence (Evansville Cancer Center); Brent Cole (Ashley Fister Cole Foundation); Colette Coyne (CCMAC); Valerie Guild (Charlie Guild Melanoma Foundation); Sue Gorham (SHADE Foundation); Drusilla Hufford (EPA), Cara Mundell (Susan Fazio

Foundation); Jean Schlipmann (The Schlip); Linda Pilkington (MRF); Catherine Poole (MIF); Kent Thornberry (Melanoma Hope Network), and many, many others. This book represents our jointly committed efforts to fight skin cancer. We shall win this fight! "Together we will find a cure for cancer not because we wished for it, but because we worked for it!"®

To John Eagleston, Margaret Merrill, and Kathleen Moncrieff, who have been with me and The Cancer Crusaders Organization from the beginning and who continuously invest (voluntarily) their limitless talents, time, energy and passion on behalf of the mission and the cause, I extend my abundant gratitude. I could not have asked for a better group of individuals to work with, and I am humbled by your compassion, commitment, and desire to serve.

To the world's best room-mates—Amy, Diane, Jenny, and Melissa, thank you. Thank you, Amy, for always making me laugh and for putting a smile on my face. Though you are still so stubborn and have yet to become a SunSavvy® girl, I know one day that you will! Diane, I admire you for your ability to speak your mind, openly, freely and articulately. Thank you, Jenny, for your quiet strength and for always slapping on the sunscreen! And, to Melissa—the sweetest, kindest, loveliest person I know. I can never thank you enough, Melissa, for always believing in me; for gently pushing me to grow and improve and therefore enabling me to progress. You always see the best in me, and, as such, have allowed me to gradually develop into a better version of myself. Thank you for your sweet, angelic and blessed friendship!

To my boss and co-workers—Jason, Jeff, Darren, Doug, Kyle, Matt, Nate, Rodney and Tom at Prosper, Inc., thanks for making it fun to come into work every day.

Thanks to five great, generous guys—Jon Bennion, John Eagleston, John Gilbert, Joseph Vogel, and Ryan Mendenhall for the encouragement. Moreover, thank you for being honorable, respectable men.

Thanks to Tim and Alaine Richards at Local Appeal for designing a fantastic book cover!

Thank you to my "critics" John Gilbert, Emily Lyons, Laurel Matsuda, and Ryan Mendenhall. Thank you for reminding me that this book was written for college students and therefore ought to be reviewed, critiqued, and edited by college students. (Hope there isn't any typos or errors).

Thanks to Amy O'Keefe and Tanya Johnson for helping transcribe more than 20 hours worth of interview tapes. Your invaluable help not only preserved my sanity but ensured the completion of this book

Thank you to Pat Benatar, Journey, Maren Ord, and Rocky IV, for providing the soundtrack to this book. Thank you for helping keep up the pace and therefore meet my publisher's deadlines.

To my favorite dermatologists, whose dedication to caring for their patients and educating their communities is truly inspiring—Dr. Elma Baron; Dr. Glen Bowen; Dr. Clay J. Cockerell; Dr. Hayes B. Gladstone; Dr. Sancy Leachman and Dr. Gregory Papadeas.

To all those who contributed to this book, especially to the families of those remembered and celebrated in this book; it is has been a joy and an honor to work with each of you. Thank you, also, to each of the dermatologists who shared their wealth of knowledge and expertise.

And, finally, to the four who inspire me most—

My Heavenly Father, I thank Thee for this unique gift called life!

My beloved mother, I pray that you can look down at me from Heaven and be proud of me. "I'll live with you forever".

My angel-friend, Melissa, if it were not for your extraordinary faith in me and for your unconditional friendship, I would never had the courage to re-do this book; I would have more than likely given up entirely. Thank you for gracing my life with your angelic presence and blessed friendship. I pray to be the friend you are to me. All my best to you, my friend, always.

To my "spirit twin"; the one who initially inspired me to do this book in the first place—Natalie. Thank you for your example of strength and courage. Thank you for trusting me with your dream of a national Skin Cancer Awareness symbol. I respect you. I appreciate you. This book is for you (and for Eric).

This book was made possible due to the generosity of Del-Ray Dermatologicals, the manufacturers of Blue Lizard Australian Suncream. Thank you for helping us serve the skin cancer community.

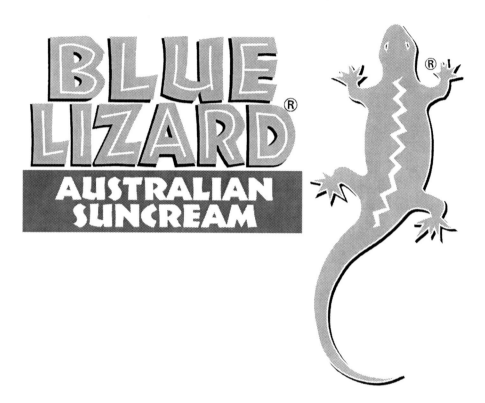

Proceeds from this distribution and circulation of this book will go to support preventing, treating, and eliminating skin cancer. To purchase additional copies, and thereby support the cause, please send an email to us at
info@cancercrusaders.org.

You may also send a tax-deductible donation to:
The Cancer Crusaders Organization
P.O. BOX 2076 Provo, Utah 84603

Foreword

Cancer has reached pandemic levels throughout the world. Well over one million new cases of skin cancers will be diagnosed this year in the United States alone. Unfortunately that number, which has been increasing yearly, is projected to continue to rise. This is due not only to the fact that many people have been exposed to dangerous ultraviolet light with inadequate protection in the past but also because individuals continue to engage in unsafe behavior such as tanning either outdoors or through the use of tanning parlors in spite of knowledge that such behavior is dangerous.

Although the skin cancer problem is quite daunting, there have been many organizations that have devoted significant time, energy and financial resources in efforts to combat it. Among these is The Cancer Crusaders Organization, founded by Danielle White. The Cancer Crusaders Organization has been the recipient of numerous awards including the prestigious Gold Triangle Award given by the American Academy of Dermatology for excellence in skin cancer education and prevention. Danielle and her organization have authored this excellent book which serves as an important resource to those who are committed to stemming the tide of skin cancer and melanoma.

I hope you find this book useful in winning the war against skin cancer.

—Clay J. Cockerell, M.D.

Dr. Cockerell is a clinical professor of dermatology and pathology and director of dermatopathology at the University of Texas Southwestern Medical Center in Dallas. He received his medical degree from Baylor College of Medicine in Houston, and completed his residency and fellowship at New York University Medical Center in New York City. He has served as secretary-treasurer and as a member of the board of directors of the American Academy of Dermatology. Dr. Cockerell served as president of the American Academy of Dermatology from 2005 until 2006. In addition, he has served as past president of the Texas Dermatological Society and of the Dallas Dermatological Society. He is the author of more than 500 publications and has served as the assistant editor of the Journal of the American Academy of Dermatology.

Preface

Trying to paint the world in orange-and-yellow Skin Cancer Awareness ribbons proves to be, for me, a double-edged sword that is both overwhelmingly challenging while all-at-once overwhelmingly rewarding, as well. Especially during the month of October when everyone is sporting all things pink in commemoration of Breast Cancer Awareness Month, therefore leaving little room for us, here at The Cancer Crusaders Organization, to wedge in our message of year-round sun safety via the utility of this new national Skin Cancer Awareness ribbon. It proves difficult, but is still very much worthwhile. It is on nights like this, when I'm staring at my computer screen, attempting to accomplish all the tasks on my lengthy "To Do List" that I find myself in earnest reflection.

At age five, I declared to my mother: "I am going to be a pediatric nurse when I grow up because I love babies and I love helping people." Four years later, at age nine, I realized that being a pediatric nurse would require that I become proficient in math, and since I loathed anything related to mathematics, I switched my career ambition to being a writer. Being a writer better suits me and my personality, anyway. I think my ninth grade honors English teacher, Mrs. Jessica Patton, explained it best by saying, "Danielle, you are the most prolific writer I know!" Indeed, I am prolific.

For sake of achieving some level of brevity, however, I reflect on the day I first heard the word "cancer", and upon my initial reluctance to be identified as a woman who lost her mother to cancer; to be a cancer crusader. I also reflect on the numerous times my professors, friends, neighbors, and fellow church members have told me over the years that I would eventually come to realize, accept, and even embrace my calling as a cancer crusader. Honestly, it wasn't until January 28, 2003, when I officially met that friend I am thinking of and praying for tonight; it wasn't until I met her that I gained a real inner strength to commit my life to this calling and to develop the faith in my Heavenly Father necessary to be guided along this "crusade". Instead of swimming among a sea of pink ribbons, as many would initially expect from me, I proudly and enthusiastically dance among orange-and-yellow ribbons partly because of the immense respect and affection I have for the person who originally created the national Skin Cancer Awareness ribbon symbol. Yet, I do it also because of the great and ever-apparent need there is in the cancer community to devote energy, time, resources, and education to combat skin cancer. The more I dedicate myself to skin cancer prevention and, in turn, come in contact with other individuals who are also crusading against this disease, I am more acutely aware of the fact that it is now part of my life's mission to combat the world's most common and preventable cancer. It is the disease that claimed the life of a gentleman I never knew but think of daily and have even grown to love; the person who inspired the creation of the national Skin Cancer Awareness symbol.

In essence, when the frustrations of coming up against the tanning industry—a $5 billion a year industry—are coupled with the lack of preventative behavior; when there is a lack of funds and support and when it feels as though I am making little or no headway are compounded, I fall to my knees in prayer. I pray for as long as my knees (and broken back) can stand it, and when I open my eyes and see that orange-and-yellow ribbon displayed in all its glory, I am again filled with strength. I am reminded of all those who are also working to provide skin cancer prevention education; all those I have grown to respect, admire, and cherish. And it is at that moment, when I am able to rise again to my feet, stand tall, and take up the call to serve.

—Danielle M. White
October 2005

From the Author

As I write this, I am sitting in the center of the food court at a local mall here in Utah. With headphones in my ear, I look up to see two 15-year-olds sitting in from me—a boy and a girl exchanging coquettish looks and stealing hugs and kisses. They are completely oblivious to the hoards of people passing them by; they are in their own little world. I turn my headphones off to take in the sounds of two giggling teenage girls to my right; I am listening to them talk about the two teenage boys sitting on my left. I am, at all once, taken back in time. I, too, am a 15-year-old girl, but I am not in the mall giggling with my best friends about boys. I am, rather, watching my mother's royal sapphire eyes gloss over black; watching a stealth predator rob me of my parent. As the dawn of New Year's morning opens its doors, it takes my mother out of it.

When I was preparing for my first Miss America franchised pageant, six years later, I initially chose a platform unrelated to cancer. A friend of mine, who at the time, was serving as Miss Utah Valley State College, urged me to seriously re-consider not choosing a cancer-related platform. "If you aren't competing for the opportunity to represent the cancer community—your passion—then why compete," she asked. "It defeats the purpose if you don't compete for a chance to serve the cancer community by being a representative for them and the cause. Do it for them. Do it for your mother. Do it for yourself. Otherwise, don't do it at all." Point taken. And so I vied for the privilege of serving the cancer community by being a representative; a voice for the cause, and therefore competed in my first Miss America franchised scholarship pageant.

Now that my "pageant days" have long since passed, I have discovered alternate forms of lending a voice to the cause and have identified ways in which I, as a 20-something single female nestled in the heart of a bustling college town, can, in my own inimitable and individualized manner, serve the cancer community. Thus, I write this, my first book.

Shall I begin with a confession? Taking on this project and writing this book has been an endless series of adventures wrought with vast emotion. Oft times I had to pause and reflect; I wondered, on numerous occasions, whether or not this book would indeed materialize from a mere idea into an actual finished product. Yet, at long last, here it is …

I am but moments away from sending the final draft to the publisher, upon which I will see the fruits of my labors.

Originally, the idea to write a book about skin cancer, and how to teach youth about it, came to me when my dear friend and co-founder, Natalie Camille Johnson, was in New York City speaking at the American Academy of Dermatology's annual Melanoma Monday Press conference. It was May 2005. Natalie was invited to share her experiences with having lost her 21-year-old brother, Eric, to complications associated with a malignant melanoma—the deadliest form of skin cancer. Yet, the subsequent series of dermatology conventions, sun safety summits, and even attending the 2005 Gold Triangle Awards and watching Natalie's dream of a universally recognized and accepted Skin Cancer Awareness symbol become a reality, left me little time to sit down and begin writing this book.

October then fell upon us. The golden sweet summer days were gone and, in their place were chills of an orange-tinted fall. October is a seemingly odd time to be re-visiting the idea of writing a book about skin cancer, but then again when you host a talk show on skin cancer/sun safety every week, it hardly seems odd at all, especially to those who know me well. They will attest to the fact that skin cancer prevention is a topic I discuss often; it is a year-round pursuit. My roommates will testify that I won't even dare step foot outside without being armed with plenty of SPF 30 sunscreen nor without a quantity of sunscreen bottles to disburse among those who cross my path. Moreover, October represents two things: national Breast Cancer Awareness month and the birth month of Natalie's brother, Eric, whom she lost to melanoma. Around this same time, I was interviewed by a student reporter from *The Daily Universe* at Brigham Young University, about my involvement with the cancer community; what inspired me to start The Cancer Crusaders Organization. One particular question was regarding my mother's passing (from breast cancer) and why I chose to fight so tenaciously for skin cancer (which claimed my co-founder's brother). "After all, it's not the disease that claimed your mother," she said. In all honesty, this is a question I am presented with often, and this time was no different, except here was this 22-year-old student reporter interviewing me on my own talk show—There I was talking live with 19 million people about why I dance among orange-and-yellow Skin Cancer Awareness ribbons and not pink ribbons for Breast Cancer Awareness, when the most important person in my life—my mother—succumbed to breast cancer.

"I have prayed about this countless times," I told her. "And I have received the same answer time and again to the point where I have no doubt that this is what my mother would want, and, more importantly, what my Heavenly Father wants for me. This is [part of] my mission." I continued further, saying "I would rather have gone in my mother's place and thus spared her life. I still have moments where I wish that He took me, and not her; however, He must have preserved my life; saved me for a very specific purpose. I believe a significant part of that is to fight this disease. And, quite frankly, isn't part of being an effective 'cancer crusader', identifying where the real immediate need is; the need that isn't currently being met or is being inadequately met, and thereby devising solutions to address that need?" I then ended the following statement:

"Fortunately, many people are already taking up the call to action and fighting for breast cancer. I am one of those people, as well. I most certainly care about fighting breast cancer for obvious reasons [but] the skin cancer community is where I really belong. It is where I feel I can contribute most and, perhaps, where I am most needed". The last question posed to me during that October 2005 interview was regarding from where, my inspiration came. "Is it your mom or is it Natalie that inspires you to be a cancer crusader?" My reply: "Both."

In truth, there was a time when I thought that could no longer continue on with this fight. One of those rare times, occurred while in the midst of writing this book. I was nearly finished when my best friend, Melissa, was anxiously anticipating being the first person to read it before sending it off to the printer. And since the publisher had asked her to write the afterword, she wanted to devour what I had written so that she can affix her official seal of approval to it and thereby publicly declare her support. Alas, I experienced a profound sense of burn-out; I was exhausted, overwhelmed. My ambition dissipated, the passion subdued. With three years of non-stop cancer crusading; proceeding forth, onward and upward, at a fastidious, relentless pace, I examined myself in the mirror one morning in early June 2006 and was forced to devote a considerable amount of time to thoughtful, honest introspection. The realization came that I needed to invest in my personal life and give time to those I love, as freely and as generously, as I had been giving to the skin cancer community. I had neglected my friends, for which (thankfully) they most understanding considering what I had been devoting my time toward—crusading. Moreover, I had been neglecting myself. I discovered that I was 27-years-old and had yet to become intimately familiar with myself; to know and like myself for simply being Danielle. Upon such a realization, I took a vacation, of sorts, and for four months I spent time enjoying the company of my friends as opposed to fretting about whether or not my book was going to be a Pulitzer worthy masterpiece. During this time, I became better acquainted with my closest friends, thereby improving and deepening our relationship, and I, for the first time, became friends with myself. I discovered that I am a multi-dimensional, multi-faceted person. With this renewed perspective, I returned to my book whereupon, something inside me broke. Ironically, in having a broader sense of perspective, a part of me was being gnawed away by fear, confusion, and inadequacy. In discovering more about myself, I became acutely aware of my faults and limitations, and different aspects about my personality that I wanted to improve upon created a strange sensation of spiritual renewal and awakening lined with pulsating pangs of self-doubt. When I returned to complete my book, after my sabbatical (keep in mind, I was still working at my "real job"), I read it only to be consumed by dissatisfaction, disappointment, even disgust. So, I expunged it. I contemplated as to how I was going to inform my partners at Del-Ray Dermatologicals, my publisher, my students, my colleagues, and my friends that I would be letting them down by failing to produce this book as promised. I wracked my brain trying to find the exact words to say to them, particularly my biggest fan, Melissa, who with her large twinkling aqua eyes had been anticipating the arrival of the <u>Only Skin Deep?® Resource Guide</u> for months as if she were but a breath away from Christmas morning. Miraculously, in the midst of searching for a way to inform everyone of my defeat, I was given a second wind. Inspired, I contracted with a new publisher, I began writing my book again, from scratch, thereby producing an exceedingly better version than previous. I believe each line of this book exudes enthusiasm, as well as my desire to serve. It is my hope those feelings pour out from the pages, warm your hearts, and inspire you to also take up the fight; to serve.

Today, I can honestly say that there are a slew of individuals who inspire me to fight on behalf of this cause. In particular, the amazing individuals featured in this book have profoundly humbled me. They have taught me the essence of courage and constantly nourish my hunger, my longing desire to serve others. If there can be a positive aspect to cancer, it is that when you dedicate yourself, and your life, to serving those touched by it, you will ultimately discover your reason for living.

You will learn that life is good; that life is beautiful. You will realize that God is good, and that the beauty of this life is that we are blessed with the ability to love and serve each other. When it is all said and done; when my Heavenly Father asks me what my favorite parts of this life were, I will, with a grateful heart shout with glee—"Thank you for allowing me to have so many people to love!" Accolades and accomplishments aside, all that I can take with me is the love I gave. Love is all we can take with us. I anxiously await the day cancer is merely a distant memory. That would be Heaven. Until then, I will, with His Grace, fight and fight to the death. And I will continue to dance among orange-and-yellow ribbons. To this end, I fight—for you.

—Danielle M. White

January 2007

Introduction

Here comes the sun—

It is more than a Beatles hit. Rather, it is a summation; a catchy lead-in, if you will, to an exploration of a rising global epidemic called skin cancer. Americans, especially, have a long-standing love affair with the sun and thus with having a "sun tan," which will contribute to more than 1.3-million new skin cancer diagnoses this year. In translation, every hour someone in America passes away from skin cancer, making it the most common of all cancers (<u>Why You Should Know About Melanoma</u>).

While commonplace, skin cancer is the most preventable cancer. The myriad affectations associated with the disease are well documented and relatively straightforward. Yet, current popular attitudes coupled with political interpretations of scientifically calculated data have the result that skin cancer fails to receive the level of activism and support that its sister, breast cancer, has been receiving. Hence, the emergence of a national Skin Cancer Awareness ribbon symbol. The ribbon, designed by my dear friend, and co-founder of The Cancer Crusaders Organization, Natalie Camille Johnson, was created in honor of her older brother, Eric, who died at age 21 of complications associated with a malignant melanoma—the deadliest form of skin cancer.

This ribbon, recently recognized by the American Academy of Dermatology with its highest honor—a Gold Triangle Award—has now been accepted as the official symbol for the cause. This first came about when Natalie and I first began working together as volunteer educators on behalf of the cancer community three years ago. Since, merging our efforts in January 2003, we extensively researched how to create a non-profit facility aimed at training young adults how to teach their peers about skin cancer prevention and sun safety, and, as such, have ceremoniously established The Cancer Crusaders Organization, which now serves as the proud home of the National Skin Cancer Awareness Symbol©.

Since acquainting the public with the National Skin Cancer Awareness Symbol© in May 2003, we have formed partnerships with various entities such as Del-Ray Dermatologicals (the manufacturers of Blue Lizard Australian Suncream), in addition to the American Academy of Dermatology's National Coalition for Sun Safety, the National Council on Skin Cancer Prevention, and the

Sun Safety Alliance. Through these partnerships we have been able to determine the level of effectives of varied promotional operations, and therefore I present this resource guide to enable you, especially young adults, to informed decisions about your dermatologic health.

First and foremost, so as to make this resource guide relevant and meaningful to individuals, particularly the college-aged population, I will utilize the first section of this book as a means of establishing a basic definition of skin cancer and thereby exploring the evolution of an (unnecessary) epidemic.

PART I

Evolution of an Epidemic

- What skin cancer is and the myriad affectations contributing to the rising skin cancer incidence

- Making a case for a universally-accepted Skin Cancer Awareness symbol

- Spotlight on Melanoma—"The Black Tumor"

Evolution of an Epidemic: Skin cancer, the world's fastest growing cancer

In a nutshell, skin cancer is a term designating the uncontrolled growth of immature cells in the skin. Each cell in the body has an internally programmed lifespan. During its lifespan the cell multiplies, replicates and divides accordingly. With a cancer cell, however, the division and replication process malfunctions; the cell fails to reach maturity and results in an "immortal" cell that eventually breaks through tissue walls and invades other normal cells. In order to better understand what skin cancer is and how it develops, examining the structure of the skin is essential.

The skin, as explained by the Dermatology Department at the University of California at Davis, is comprised of an outer layer called the epidermis which has a depth of only about 20 cells making it equivalent to the thickness of a sheet of paper. Below this layer lies the "dermis" containing tiny blood and lymph vessels, which increase as the skin gets deeper. Cells called melanocytes are found in the transitional layer between the epidermis and dermis. These skin cells, called melanin, or pigmentation, help to protect against the damaging rays of the sun and determine skin coloring and proliferate into moles or "spots."

Three types of skin cancer can be distinguished. The two most common forms, also known as non-melanoma skin cancer, are basal cell carcinoma and squamous cell carcinoma. The final and most life-threatening skin cancer is melanoma because it has a high propensity to metastasize ("spread") to other organs in the body if not detected early. A melanoma arises in the melanocytes, which, again, are the cells that produce the melanin responsible for pigmentation. In fact, damaged melanin by exposure to ultraviolet is what causes the skin to become red from "sun burn." According to Melanoma International, melanomas develop initially as a flat phase without competence for metastasis which is also referred to as the radial growth phase. Melanomas may, however, evolve during a vertical growth phase and become elevated with a tendency to spread.

Unlike most cancers, melanoma is said to ordinarily derive from external environmental factors as opposed to hereditary or familial links. Researchers at the Huntsman Cancer Institute (HCI) however, are extensively analyzing to what extent genetic factors play into one's likeliness of having a melanoma. Sancy A. Leachman, M.D., Ph.D., deputy director at the Tom C. Mathews Jr. Familial Melanoma Research Clinic at Huntsman Cancer Institute, and a professor of dermatology at the University of Utah, reports that persons with numerous dysplastic nevi (abnormal moles)—a largely hereditary issue—do appear to possess a risk for future melanomas. Yet, Dr. Leachman, who also sits on boards for the American Academy of Dermatology (AAD), asserts, as do a number of other medical professionals, that the extent of sun exposure a person sustains during their first 18 years of life proves to be a more conclusive risk. Therefore, she confirms the aforementioned statement that skin cancer is unique in that it is largely induced by external environmental factors, such as excessive UV exposure, rather than inherited gene mutations, such as p16. Though, familial factors do a play a part in one's risk skin cancer.

According to National and Aeronautics Space Administration (NASA), the use of "external environmental factors" refers to ozone depletion and the subsequent increase in ultraviolet irradiation and exposure, which has circumstantially contributed to at least 90% of skin carcinomas. Coinciding with NASA findings, the Environmental Protection Agency (EPA) has reported that, as of September 2003, the earth's ozone has a hole equivalent to the size of North America that will result in an estimated 40 million skin cancer incidents, worldwide, in 2007. In effect, scientists at the National Research Council say that just a 10% global loss of ozone results in a minimum 26% increase in skin cancer incidence meaning that a 1% decrease in ozone layer triples the increase in UV irradiation (Human Health Effects). The severity of the ozone-sun exposure relationship is demonstrated by the fact that 70 years ago the probability of a person living in the United States of developing a melanoma was 1 in 1,500, as compared to today's 1 in 65. It is projected, by the NRC, that 1 in 50 persons will have a melanoma in 2007. In other words, an American's lifetime risk for melanoma is 1 in 5 (Aric 37).

In conjunction with researchers at the National Research Council, NASA engineers continually investigate ozone depletion, its ripple effect of increased ultraviolet radiation secretion and its role in skin carcinomas, especially the aggrandized, and oftentimes fatal malignant melanoma. Researchers say that "The much more dangerous malignant melanoma is not as well understood [as basal cell or squamous cell carcinomas]. [However] there appears to be a correlation between brief, high intensity exposure to UV and eventual appearance—as long as 10-to-20 years—of melanoma. Twice as many deaths due to melanomas are seen in Utah, Texas, and Florida" (<u>Health Effects of UV-B Light</u>). The mentioning of Utah is exceptionally pertinent because Utah's risk is the highest in the nation—1 in 52 versus 1 in 65 nationally, according to HCI. A combination higher land elevation (hence, a closer proximity to shorter UV-A and UV-B wavelengths), along with a relatively large population of fairer-skinned citizens contributes to the 500+ incidences of skin cancer incidence in Utah and Colorado each year, as reported by the American Cancer Society.

A plethora of scientific, medical, and even sociological journals share the same sentiment regarding UV-A and UV-B rays as an integral element in an individual's potential for skin cancer. Various studies on DNA and how UV irradiation plays an effectual role explain how excessive sun exposure dramatically affects DNA structures leading to skin cancers.

DNA damage due to UV exposure depends on the level of duration, as well as the susceptibility and resilience of the exposed organism. The toll UV irradiation takes on human health include: skin cancer, cataracts, and the weakening of one's immune system response. And while sunlight acts as a catalyst in the generation of vitamin D "large amounts of UV-B [and UV-A], however, are harmful to a wide range of biological systems" (Scotto 1333). John Scottery of <u>Scientific American</u> online puts it this way, saying that a consequence of damage to DNA molecules in the skin from UV rays is the synthesis of different proteins and enzymes: "The effects of these proteins, notably prostaglandins and cytokines, lead to dilation of the cutaneous blood vessels and recruitment of inflammatory cells." Scottery continues, "The body does have mechanisms to repair damaged DNA after ultraviolet exposure. But as the frequency of sunlight exposure increases, so, too, does the probability [of a future skin cancer diagnosis]." In sum, DNA absorbs ultraviolet light which sequentially can break bonds of DNA. Unrepaired genetic damage deriving from the absorption of ultra-violet radiation energy frequently leads to either an actual skin cancer diagnosis or at least a heightened risk for such diagnosis. As a result of this augmented exposure to UV rays united with higher land elevation, there is a continually higher-than-average skin cancer mortality rate particularly in Utah where there more than 224 days of sunshine, according to the University of Utah Department of Dermatology. The ACE Foundation and Skin Cancer Foundation, perhaps sum it up best by saying, "The risk of developing a malignant melanoma is directly related to the sensitivity of an individual's skin to the sun" (Aric 37). Residents of Utah especially, possess many of the risk factors associated with this mentioned sun sensitivity such as fair skin, blonde or red hair, and blue or green eyes. Alas, no one is immune from the risk of skin cancer. Consider the infamous Reggae singer Bob Marely of Jamaica, for instance. Marley passed away from complications associated with a malignant melanoma that metastized into his lungs and brain, at age 36.

Despite a heightened risk due to external environmental factors, proven effective preventative measures exist to facilitate a combative stance against skin cancer. These proven prevention measures include proper use of sunscreens along with a sun protection factor (SPF) of at least 15, wearing wide-brimmed hats and long sleeves, and UV protective sunglasses, avoiding direct sunlight—year round—between the hours of 10:00 a.m. and 4:00 p.m., and performing monthly skin exams (<u>Why You Should Know About Melanoma</u>). Challenging to skin cancer prevention education efforts, however, is the disparity in awareness and action stimulated as a by-product of popular culture. A review of several studies demonstrates this disparity.

In June 2003, the Centers for Disease Control and Prevention (CDC) conducted a survey in partnership with the American Academy of Dermatology, of 1,001 Americans ages 18-to-24 to determine their level of understanding about melanoma. The survey indicates that approximately 50% of men and 35% of women did not recognize the term "melanoma." The younger survey participants demonstrated the least amount of melanoma skin cancer awareness. Correspondingly, participants were generally able to correctly identify the early warning signs of melanoma, only about 58% knew that just one severe childhood sunburn was "an established risk factor in the development of melanoma later in life" (<u>Prevention of Skin Cancer by Reducing Exposure</u>). Also noteworthy is that sustaining even just one severe "blistering or peeling" sunburn prior to age 18 increases one's potential for a future melanoma by a minimum of 60%, according to the National Cancer Institute. A similar such study conducted in June 2005 echoes much of the same. According to the Sun Safety Alliance, 85% of Americans know the dangers of over-exposure to ultraviolet radiation, and the subsequent increase in risk for skin cancer; however only 56% take measures to protect their skin from the sun. (*Sunscreen Use Down as Skin Cancer rates Increase*). "Motivating people is key," says Phil Schneider, executive director of the Sun Safety Alliance. "These numbers clearly demonstrate that public awareness is not translating into action."

Evolution of an Epidemic: Making a case for Skin Cancer Awareness

For reasons previously mentioned, The Cancer Crusaders Organization recently conducted a random survey of 500 college students (ages 17-to-30) in Utah, Tennessee, and Massachusetts, as a means of analyzing melanoma knowledge by this primary target public. Responses generated were akin to those generated by the original CDC survey; only 181 of the 500 polled report being familiar with term "melanoma" thus re-emphasizing the need and importance of efficiently crafted prevention education mediums for this primary target public. Cleverly packaged and marketable awareness campaigns such as the "Sun Guy" by Crow-ell Advertising for the Utah Cancer Control Program, do appear to achieve a level of success in familiarizing the public with skin cancer. Nevertheless, to claim that an elevated consciousness and comprehension alone will suffice is to ignore that there remains a disparity between awareness and action despite such campaigns. Problematic are societal attitudes and behaviors.

This scenario is well depicted through a study directed by Ingrid Taylor from the University of British Columbia. Taylor interviewed 175 patients in August 2003 questioning them about seeking attention for skin lesions which were later diagnosed as malignant melanoma. She found that even patients having a good, basic melanoma knowledge and its relationship with sun exposure still delayed obtaining prompt medical attention and did not decrease their level of sun exposure. Taylor reports, "It's not enough that people know about risks, we need to find a way to change their behavior" (<u>Prevention of Skin Cancer by Reducing Exposure</u>).

Reiterating Taylor's study is another conducted by Dr. Mona Saraiya of the Task Force on Community Prevention Services with the CDC. In the September 2003 online edition of the *Guide to Community Preventive Services*, Saraiya points out that systematically reviewed evidence based on recommendations by health professionals, environmental activists, and mass media outlets revealed that more than 50% of Americans fail to sufficiently protect themselves from harmful UV rays. She continues, "While knowledge of the risk of sun exposure and the use of sunscreens and other forms of sun protection have improved over the past two decades, a gap still exists between knowledge and behavior."

Therefore, after reviewing more than 6,200 journal titles, 216 articles, and 97 studies, I must pose the question: What are the most effective strategies to encourage and improve skin cancer prevention behavior? Through my experiences as a skin cancer educator, I believe that the personalized approach seems more relevant to the public—more relevant than spouting scientific jargon. Such a personalized approach makes it possible for the instructor to reach his or her public on multiple levels and has proven, time and again, to be among those effective strategies.

As a trained skin cancer educator, and host of an award-winning radio and television talk show on skin cancer—*"Conversations with Cancer"*—I speak to an estimated 19 million individuals every week across the globe via internet broadcasts. Furthermore, I speak to roughly 75 people every week at various seminars, conferences, and events. Through this, I have witnessed first-hand how the formation of intimate connections vastly shapes the audience. In attendance at the majority of these seminars are women's groups, skin care consultants, students, and support coalitions. When I speak and present, I include the distinctive perspective of having lost my mother (and many friends) to cancer. In addition, for the last 12 years I have also worked with cancer patients one-on-one. Both of these personal perspectives furnish a much-needed human touch. Almost instanteously, I am transformed from an instructor to an advocate, a neighbor, and a peer. In metamorphising from "talking head" into a friend, I am able to gain a level of trust through transmitting that we are all vulnerable to cancer, but at the same time emphasizing that it is indeed possible to triumph. Consequently, my audience feels empowered.

On a daily basis I am presented with opportunity of being approached by at least one individual who will openly divulge the details of his or her experience with skin cancer. Whether the experience is direct or through a loved one, individuals plead with me to be their mouthpiece. Recently, as a result of these requests, I have come into a sharper, stark realization for the need to lobby to community and political leaders to prompt them to act on behalf of cancer prevention and to inspire their constituents to follow suit.

We, at The Cancer Crusaders Organization, based on survey findings and personal experiences, have determined that specifically delivered media interventions designed to increase knowledge and awareness influence attitude, beliefs, and intentions, are also among the best methods of communication—especially with regard to the college-age population. As participants in the execution of a variety of promotions and campaigns we find that successful mediums which are typically low-intensity (or "less effective") include CD-ROM based kiosks and UV index reports in newspapers. Higher-intensity, more effective tools include television commercials, billboards, interactive educational programs, and face-to-face communication.

We present then, not a challenge of fostering a value for educational instruction amongst our target public; rather, we relay information to our audience in a manner that specifically keys into their self-interests and the interests of people around them. For example, consider how society is largely driven by appearances and how ideals associated with appearances have enabled those in the tanning industry to have a phenomenal stronghold influence on so-called modernity. Consider how concentrated mediums have propelled and perpetuated ideals that define and constitutes "healthy" or "beautiful" and how those ideals have saturated our culture.

The Indoor Tanning Association (ITA), which represents owners of tanning booths and salons, recently criticized a joint study conducted by the Food and Drug Administration, the AAD, and the CDC in September 2003 stating the dangers associated with tanning and malignant melanomas. Dan Humiston, ITA president, denounced the claims made in the study that there are connections between deadly skin cancer and exposure from tanning beds. Yet, Dr. Elizabeth Whitmore of the American Academy of Dermatology says, "People continue to invest both time and money to visit tanning salons despite evidence which have found an increased incidence of melanoma [...] in those who visit indoor tanning salons" (Whitmore). Joyce Ayoub, director of public information at the Skin Cancer Foundation, agrees with the AAD, saying "Any tan means damage to the skin." With this, however, the indoor tanning industry continues to be highly profitable (yielding nearly $5 billion in annual revenues) as a result of mainstream cultural attitudes that to be tan is to be fashionable. She agrees that pop icons play a significant role in these ideas of attractiveness.

In illustrating these conceptual ideas of attractiveness, consider how American definitions of "beauty" are in constant state of modification. Today the media inundates society with images of a blonde and bronze Charlize Theron, "Best Actress" Academy Award Winner for her role in *Monster*. In contrast, the ideal picture of femininity in the 1930s was Vivien Leigh, "Best Actress" Academy Award Winner for her role as Scarlett O'Hara in *Gone With The Wind,* whose porcelain skin gave her an elegant and regal, if not statuesque presence. Clearly, ideals have dramatically changed, as demonstrated by Charlize (in the photo below) who, like a myriad other female actresses, models, and figureheads, opt for the popular "tanning glow." If only our youth would adhere to the advice given by professional volleyball player, Gabrielle Reece, who, in her best-selling book Big Girl In The Middle, said "Attractiveness is all in your way of being" (Reece 65). Reece continues, later on in her book to say that "I would like to represent someone who, regardless of the degree of support, listens to her own voice instead of trying to conform to a bunch of societal rules that change every five or 10 years anyway" (Reece 231).

Furthermore, the degree of influence the tanning industry has on society is seen through a report issued by the National Cancer Institute (NCI) in conjunction with Cancer-Wise in May 2002 that indicates, nearly a third of Caucasian teenage girls in America have used a tanning bed at least three times. In a series of surveys conducted over a period of four years by The Cancer Crusaders Organization, we learned that of the 1-million high school and college students we interviewed and surveyed over the past four years, nearly 90% of them said they have tanned at least once in their lifetime, and nearly half continue to do so despite being apprised of the risks for skin cancer. Perhaps, even more concerning are results generated from a survey conducted by the American Academy of Dermatology in May 2005. The American Academy of Dermatology discovered that the popularity of tanning beds among teenagers has only increased. Nearly 70% of young adults, aged 18-to-23, reported that despite knowing someone who has skin cancer, they remained un-deterred from frequenting tanning salons.

During our first skin cancer prevention education conference as an incorporated non-profit organization held in spring 2004 at Utah Valley State College, we offered free skin screenings, question and answer sessions, as well as an instructional PowerPoint presentation. More than 60 students attended the presentation, and another 125 students participated in the skin screenings and question-and-answer sessions. One of the students that attended the event made the following comment to dermatologist Anneli Bowen, M.D., from the University of Utah School of Medicine: "The problem is, now that we know that tanning and too much sun exposure is harmful and can cause skin cancer, there is still an urge to be golden." Again, the challenge is modifying attitudes so that individuals, especially the college-aged population, will act in accordance to the knowledge they have gleaned from these skin cancer prevention education presentations.

Thus, only until we key into the self-interests of these young adults, their lack of behavioral responses will only further contribute to ever-increasing number of skin cancer-related deaths. We must express, if not stress, that while they are seeking the coveted "bronze look" their pursuits are ultimately defeating, for not only are they significantly increasing their risk for melanoma skin cancer, they are expediting the aging process; their skin is aging prematurely as a result of this incessant exposure to ultraviolet radiation. Moreover, we must also enlighten to them to the fact that prevention not only enhances the overall quality of life in America, but it is far less expensive than treatment. America spends more than $50 million annually treating cancer and an additional $44 billion in direct medical expenses associated with cancer (McCarthy). In fact, according to the World Health Organization, the global cost of cancer treatment exceeded $190 billion last year. As a result of considering data obtained through research and the combined first-hand experience we have, I have also examined how two very different causes achieved wide spread success in rallying awareness and support. In doing this, we are better equipped to design and market the new national Skin Cancer Awareness ribbon and recognize that, indeed, it is public perspective that immensely influences the discrepancy in Skin Cancer Awareness versus Breast Cancer Awareness. Consider the emergence of the Breast Cancer Awareness movement and how breast cancer activists have been able to gain significant recognition for their pink ribbon symbol, and likewise with the AIDS movement for their red ribbon symbol.

Almost before the first leaf is painted orange by October fall, a slew of companies mass produce cartons, lids, and other such packaging paraphernalia inked with pretty pink. It is "Breast Cancer Awareness Month" and whether you know someone who has been affected by this disease or not, you are aware of what a pink ribbon represents. You may even be more inclined to purchase bottles of Yoplait yogurt simply for the sake of having $.10 of that purchase go towards the cause. Behold, the power of pink. This almost universal recognition; however, did not come about without years of rallying.

The materialization of the pink Breast Cancer Awareness ribbon has origins in the feminist movement of the 1960s when women were encouraged to become more empowered. Being proactive about health care options and the maintenance of their bodies were surrounded by the many and vast issues associated with this time. Nevertheless, it was not until the mid-1980s when a different group of activists came together to adopt a symbol and therefore heighten awareness of its particular crusade: AIDS.

The red ribbon for AIDS took effect seemingly without delay and circled throughout the globe, making it acceptable to acknowledge the epidemic and the need for action. More than 20 years later—both the red and pink ribbons have become a virtually universal and systematic tool for putting a face to the respective disease each represent. So effective is the pink Breast Cancer Awareness ribbon, in particular, that numerous research facilities dedicated to cancer-related issues use it in every state across the country. The American Cancer Society, which was traditionally the basic, primary source for cancer education and aid, is now merely a modem feeding into mass channels in a feverish pursuit of a cure. Praise to the pink ribbon that has championed breast cancer.

As Ellen J. Reifler, a columnist for Herizon magazine relates, "It is an understandable leap in logic for those concerned about breast cancer to think that, like many tactics of the AIDS activists, ribbons would work for us. A sea of pink ribbons, all signifying the solidarity with the cause, would seem to be just the ticket" (Reifler 26). While Reifler is not completely convinced or confident that pink is entirely appropriate for initiating an "I will not be silenced" stance, she does acknowledge that "For some advocates wearing a pink ribbon signifies that women with or without breast cancer [...] don't need to fear this disease" (Reifler 26). In other words, the pink ribbon conveys a need for hope. It must also be acknowledged that the purpose of a pink ribbon is not solely for fighting cancer itself. Breast cancer encompasses not only the disease, but also the actual woman as a human being, the woman's family and friends, and the woman's health care provider. The ribbon symbol is a tool for everyone touched by cancer to various depths and degrees.

The concept of a ribbon symbol is not merely a marvel of marketing at its optimum best, but it is an avenue. A visual aid, it allows people to identify with the cause on an interpersonal but non-intrusive level. It portrays the cancer as real, as opposed to this elusive, intangible and outwardly unconquerable foe. Proclaiming that the pink Breast Cancer Awareness ribbon is a means for women who suffer from the disease to be remembered is apparent and for that reason it succeeds in its objective and its function to raise awareness. Akin to yellow ribbons Americans wear during times of war and conflict to honor soldiers abroad (or to represent Teen Suicide Awareness); the pink Breast Cancer Awareness ribbon is worn to honor patients, families, and communities.

It is this very notion of empowerment which spawns hope. It is why Natalie and I, and our fellow cancer crusaders, feel that having a national ribbon symbol for Skin Cancer Awareness is vital to the campaign.

Natalie chose to implement a sunburst in the center of the ribbon to represent how sun exposure plays an integral part in skin cancer incidence, and the orange is representative of October—the birth month of her late brother Eric. While many cancers have a colored ribbon symbol, such as the gold-trimmed ribbon for lung cancer, the blue ribbon for prostate cancer, and the purple ribbon for pancreatic cancer, black was once unofficially used for melanoma. Black, we feel, is inappropriate. Black does not espouse hope. The new and official national Skin Cancer Awareness ribbon has been designed to espouse hope, in addition to conveying an accurate portrait of the inter-relational link between sun exposure and increasing skin cancer incidence. Thusly the ribbon employs effective colors in its design. After establishing the right look and feel into the ribbon design prototype, Natalie presented her original design for a universal symbol to the National Coalition for Sun Safety, at the American Academy of Dermatology, and, through our combined efforts, we have gained and secured positive support for the symbol introducing it to more than 400,000,000 people across the globe, as of January 1, 2007, via our award-winning *"Only Skin Deep?"*® Skin Cancer Prevention Campaign which serves as a launch pad towards further introducing the Skin Cancer Awareness ribbon, and for implementing effective educational programs such as our "ONLY SKIN DEEP?"® Peer Educator's Training & Certification Program.

Granted, merely heightening one's awareness to this all too common, and very preventable disease, is not enough. Yet, the National Skin Cancer Awareness Symbol©, in its effective visual representation of the cause at-hand, is a key; a launch pad, if you will, that helps reiterate the crusader's rally cry: *We can conquer this disease! We will find a cure!* The motto we have embraced at The Cancer Crusaders Organization is "Together we will find a cure to cancer not because we wished for it but because we worked for it." The ribbon creates a visual—puts a face to the disease. It affirms that there are real people who suffer—directly or indirectly. It avows that we must fight. And so we shall.

Evolution of an Epidemic: Spotlight on Melanoma—"The Black Tumor"

Known in the time of Hippocrates as "The Black Tumor", melanoma is an especially unique type of cancer in a variety of ways. The first, and perhaps, most obvious reason being that you can actually "see" it. Melanoma is, often times, visible on your skin; however, do not be mislead by its visibility factor. Melanomas can, and often do, burrow deep beneath the skin with a high likeliness for spreading into the lymphnodes and other bodily organs. Melanoma is also inimitable when compared to the other skin cancers, in that it is a separate and distinct form of skin cancer. While basal cell carcinomas and squamous cell carcinomas share common characteristics and even links, melanoma does not. It is in a class all by itself. What also makes melanoma extraordinary, is its extremely aggressive nature. Melanoma is the deadliest form of skin cancer. It is not our objective to frighten you by saying this, yet it is imperative that we be completely honest and forthright. Melanoma is quite dangerous, especially if not detected and treated while in its early stages. Furthermore, melanoma incidence and mortality has radically been increasing over the last century. In just the last year, the American Academy Dermatology and the American Cancer Society have reported a 10% increase in melanoma incidence. It is estimated that 105,750 new cases of melanoma will be diagnosed in 2007, with nearly 8,000 of those resulting in death. Melanoma actually accounts for over 75% of skin cancer deaths. Putting the seriousness of this disease into perspective, melanoma is now the most common cancer among women ages 20-to-29, and the leading cause of cancer death among women ages 25-to-45. Melanoma is even being seen in elementary school children. One of our partners has a young son, just 12-years-old, who was recently diagnosed with melanoma.

With that, one may ask "But what *is* melanoma? I need to understand it before I can prevent it." If we dissect the term melanoma in half, we end up with the two words—"mela" and "noma". The root "mela" comes from the word melanocytes, which are the cells in your skin responsible for pigmentation. The latter half of the term, "noma" comes from the word carcinoma which is a term referring to cancers of the body's external tissues, such as the skin. In sum, melanoma is the cancer of the melanocytes in your skin.

Melanoma is not a respecter of persons. Everyone is at risk for getting melanoma. As discussed in previously, individuals of fair-skinned races do appear to be at greater risk for developing melanoma than those of darker-skinned races, but anyone can get melanoma. In the United States, alone, Caucasians are 20 times more likely to develop melanoma than African-Americans. Worldwide, fair-skinned (or Caucasian) populations have the highest risk of developing melanoma. Interestingly enough, Asian populations have the lowest risk for getting melanoma. Yet, it is possible for anyone, with skin, to get melanoma.

Here in the United States we have experienced a dramatic increase in the number of melanoma cases over the past 20 years. According to the American Cancer Society, the incidence rate for melanoma (number of new cases of melanoma per 100,000 people each year) has more than doubled since 1973. Summarily, 1 in 34 Americans have a lifetime risk of developing melanoma during their lifetime; an American's lifetime risk is 1 in 5.

Conversely, the world's highest incidence of melanoma is in Australia, which has a sizeable fair-skinned immigrant population. Melanoma is the most common malignancy in Australia. On that same note, however, Australians are now beginning to see a marginal decrease in the average number of Stage IV malignant melanomas which has been largely attributed to Australia's extensive, and comprehensive, skin cancer screening and educational programs.

Melanoma, though distinctive, does develop in a manner similar to other cancers. Damage to DNA causes cells to divide and grow without control or order, eventually becoming a malignant tumor. The first malignant tumor diagnosed as melanoma usually develops atop the skin. Yet, if not caught in its early stages, melanoma will grow and spread along the epidermis before penetrating deep into the dermis and eventually coming into contact with lymph and blood vessels.

To provide you with a better understanding of how a mole can become cancerous, let us quickly review a few items we learned in Biology 101. A skin lesion is any type of skin growth, regardless of whether it is benign (non-cancerous) or malignant (cancerous). Moles are clusters of melanocytes (cells responsible for producing pigmentation or melanin) that form pigmented spots on the skin. The most common are moles and freckles. The medical term for mole is nevus (nevi for plural), which is the Latin word for birthmark. Ordinary moles are usually a uniform brown, tan, or flesh-colored spot and smaller than six millimeters, or 1/4 inch, in diameter, the width of a pencil eraser. Moles may emerge anywhere on the skin, either singly or in a group. Several moles may appear on the skin at the same time, especially in areas that have been exposed to the sun. Once a mole has developed, its size, shape, and color tend to change slightly over time. Everyone has moles and other related growths on their skin. For some, including myself, we have numerous moles—both benign and dysplastic. As mentioned before, most of these "spots" are birthday presents, meaning they are congenital; we were born with them. Yet, we also acquire moles as we grow into adulthood. It is important to know that while some skin lesions may resemble melanoma, many of them, in actuality, are benign growths and are harmless and remain stable throughout our lifespan. On occasion, however, new growths may develop and previous moles may undergo change. These lesions may signal skin cancer, or be precursors of skin cancer, even melanoma—the deadliest form of skin cancer. Thus it imperative we closely monitor our skin through monthly self-skin exams and annual visits to the dermatologist.

Fortunately, by becoming acutely familiar with your own skin; knowing what is considered "normal" for your skin, you will be better able to distinguish between those normal growths and those requiring immediate evaluation by your favorite board certified dermatologist (preferably one that specializes in skin cancer). With that established, it is imperative you are able to recognize changes in a mole that may suggest that a melanoma is developing. The first sign of melanoma is **change**. Any change in the size, shape, or color of an existing mole or the appearance of a new mole. More commonly, though, melanomas are found in an area where a new mole-like pigmentation has appeared. If you notice changes in a mole (or see a suspicious new mole), contact your dermatologist immediately! If you do not have a dermatologist, get a complete list of dermatologists, who are board certified and in good standing with the American Academy of Dermatology, by logging on to www.aad.org. Perhaps, the most crucial, essential component in protecting yourself from skin cancer, especially melanoma, is becoming an active, informed patient. In other words, be your own best advocate. This will, in turn, inevitably assist your dermatologist with providing you the best care. This is what Part II of this book is all about—building an open, honest relationship with your dermatologist so as to reduce your likeliness of a future skin cancer diagnosis.

PART II

A) Building a Relationship with the Dermatologist; Empowering Patients

- Choosing a dermatologist that is right for you and preparing the initial visit

- Understanding the both the role of a dermatologist and patient in reducing your risk

- Fostering and facilitating effective communication between dermatologist and patient

- Understanding your melanoma risk

- Coping with a skin cancer diagnosis

- Treatment options and procedures

B) Finding Effective Sun Protection

- The basics of preventing the most preventable cancer

- -Choosing a sunscreen and how to maximize its efficacy

- Making a real fashion statement with sun protective clothing

Choosing a Dermatologist and Preparing for the Initial Visit

Last summer my room-mate, Jenny, invited all four of us, her fellow room-mates, us to her parents' house for Sunday dinner. When introductions were being made, Jenny mentioned that I run a non-profit organization and that the orange- and-yellow ribbon pin on my lapel was [is] the official Skin Cancer Awareness symbol. There began a lengthy discussion on one of my favorite topics—skin cancer prevention, which no less failed to surprise my other room-mates who have now grown quite accustomed to my impassioned sermons on the impor- tance of skin cancer prevention. Yet, ever-patient and supportive room-mates were likely surprised to find the casual chatter of a Sunday gathering turn into an intellectual discussion that delved deep into the importance of building a rela- tionship with your dermatologist. One of the gentleman there, Jenny's towering 6'7" brother-in-law; an outdoor enthusiast and father of three young children, approached me, quietly, while helping clear the table—"Danielle, I have had four family members die of melanoma." I asked him, "Have you ever gone up to the Tom C. Mathews Jr. Familial Melanoma Research Clinic at Huntsman Cancer Institute in Salt Lake and been thoroughly screened and assessed? Do you have a dermatologist that you see every year? Who is your dermatologist? I might know them and we can make up a list of questions, together, for you to ask during your next visit." This towering, stocky man, with a voice so powerful and command- ing it reverberated within me, almost embarrassingly replied "Woah! Slow down there for a minute, Danielle! I mean, my mom used to nag me to get this ugly mole on back cut off, but I haven't actually been in to see a dermatologist to have my skin checked out much less find out what my melanoma risk is or get medical advice." By this time, our fellow room-mate—my best friend—Melissa, the Texas-raised ballerina with blemish-free porcelain skin, corn silk blonde hair, and aquamarine eyes, had put down her dish rag to lean over my shoulder and listen intently. "Can you believe this girl," says the brother-in-law, John, to the newest member of our conversation, Melissa. "Is she always this concerned about mak- ing sure people go to the dermatologist?" Melissa's reply: "Yep, she sure is.

Danielle doesn't just tell you to protect yourself she teaches you *how* to protect yourself. So, speaking of that, I'm curious about these questions we should be asking the dermatologist because my dad is outside cleaning pools all day, getting so much sun he looks as though he's of a different race, and I want to know how I can encourage him to go in and get his skin checked out by a dermatologist." That, then, initiated an impromptu lesson on how to build a relationship with your dermatologist. After about 10 minutes of list making, several of the other family members joined in with additional questions and points of concern. I had to chuckle at men, with their reluctance, were asking me ways they can, essentially, by-pass or even avoid going into the dermatologist, whereas all of the women were asking me about the best tricks to coax the men. "How do I get my husband in to see the dermatologist without having to deal with his whining and without it having to be a constant battle or struggle?" To this, Melissa, replied:

"Anything worthwhile takes work, and building relationships are not meant to be easy. It takes constant effort. It takes a lot of work [but] when you invest in building [and maintaining] relationships you find that both [parties involved] are blessed." Melissa continued on to say, "This is essentially the same thing that Danielle is saying when she talks about having a good relationship with your dermatologist being the first crucial step in protecting yourself [...] from having to deal with a skin cancer later on in the future. Anything worthwhile requires a real personal effort. Relationships are no exception." To be honest, I could scarcely hide my emotion. My eyes became wet with tears. I could feel myself, quite literally, beaming with pride and joy. It is in moments such as this, when I think that, perhaps, all the tenacious effort and persistent praying that young adults "get the message", does, indeed, make a difference and that it does impact people for the better. Well, at least in this particular instance it did make a difference. All the many hours of "preaching" sun safety that have taken place within the walls of our tiny college apartment equipped Melissa with ability to drive the message home to Jenny's seemingly indestructible brother-in-law, John, and convinced him to promise us, most importantly his wife, that he would call the dermatologist we recommended. John even asked me if I could recommend any books or pieces of educational literature he should read before paying a visit to the dermatologist. I referred him to the official Web-site of the American Academy of Dermatology and reviewed the "In Preparation For My First Visit List" we collaborated on together, which included a list of materials he should bring with him to the dermatologist (e.g., medical records, a tape recorder and notebook), questions he should ask, even questions his wife should ask, and a list of common medical terms the dermatologist may use when describing the signs and symptoms of skin cancer.

Albeit, before continuing any further, it is imperative to provide a real life case-in-point illustrating the value in not only forming a relationship with your dermatologist, but, moreover, becoming your own best advocate. Consider the story of Bob Marley. We mentioned him briefly earlier in this book; however, learning of Bob Marely's battle with melanoma provides a poignant picture of how crucial it is to take an active role in your own health.

Contrary to popular belief Bob Marley did not die of a drug overdose, rather he was diagnosed with malignant melanoma which spread into his lungs and brain. This factoid might surprise a few readers, but melanoma is not restricted to "white people only". This piece of information should actually bring the seriousness of this disease into a shaper, more stark perspective. Bob Marley's battle with melanoma is a noteworthy case-and-point.

Bob Marley's melanoma was first thought to have been an old soccer injury. The wound on his right big toe, which was originally found in July 1977, proved problematic after months of lingering ulceration. The wound simply would not heal. It was then that the correct diagnosis of malignant melanoma was made by doctors. And the melanoma appeared to be growing, aggressively, under his toenail. Marley was advised to get his toe amputated, but he refused because of deeply held religious beliefs (he was Rastafarian) He also was concerned about the impact such an operation would have on his dancing. He felt that amputation "would profoundly affect his career at a time when greater success was close at hand" according to biographers. Sadly, Bob Marley's melanoma spread to his brain, his lungs and his stomach. While on tour in the summer of 1980, while trying to break into the U.S. market, he collapsed while jogging in Central Park (New York). Marley did seek alternative advice regarding his melanoma diagnosis, but it was to no avail. He died a year later on May 11, 1981. He was just 36-years-old and at the peak of his music career. If we learn anything from Bob Marley's story, it is that no one is exempt from a melanoma diagnosis. Moreover, we learn that taking action on anything of concern is imperative. Do not be afraid to "listen to your body" and do not be afraid to open your mouth; ask questions and seek help from your dermatologist. After all, you are your own best advocate. Bob Marley dismissed an unrelenting sore on his toe as a stubborn soccer injury, for which he paid the ultimate price—his life. In that, I implore everyone take a pro-active position in protecting yourself from skin cancer. You owe it to yourself, and to those who love you, to do so.

That being said, over the span of nine months (between July 2005 and March 2006), I interviewed several respected dermatologists, considered by the American Academy of Dermatology to be leading experts in the prevention, detection, and treatment of skin cancer. I have, with their permission, incorporated excerpts from these interviews in to this section so as to emphasis the great importance of developing two-way communication with your dermatologist and hence becoming your own best advocate

The first time I visited a dermatologist was as a 19-year-old who had just moved from California to Utah to attend Brigham Young University and was particularly perturbed with the fact that her skin not only developed a severe case of eczema, but that her acne became "out of control" and nothing was working to clear it up nor remedy it. I kept thinking to myself—*How is it that my acne is 10 times worse now, than it ever was in high school?* So, determined to resolve this acne that was now taking over my body, I looked for dermatologists in the yellow pages—looking for one that was within walking distance. Upon finding a dermatologist in close proximity from my apartment, I inquired about the cost—"It is $80.00 just to be seen," said a high-pitched voice on the other end of the phone. *$80.00 just to be seen! Well, I hope my utilities will be cheap this month!* And thus I proceeded to book the appointment. Three weeks later, I went in to the dermatologist's office. While there, I, briefly, made mention of my moles; should it concern me that I have so many moles? Both of my parents had a lot of moles. Is that of any significance? Much to my dismay (especially now that I know better) the dermatologist did not address the issue of my numerous dysplastic nevi. Because I had scheduled an appointment to discuss my severe acne and to treat my eczema, that is what he addressed. And there ended the discussion and the appointment. I tried the atopical treatments he prescribed, the acne cleared up (for the most part) and the eczema disappeared. It would be five years before I visited the dermatologist again.

Needless to say, the next time I visited a dermatologist was as the result of befriending a [former] Miss Utah by the name of Natalie Camille Johnson. I was competing in pageants, at that time, as part of the Miss America Scholarship Program, and had been told, repeatedly, that I "just had to meet Natalie Johnson!" After competing in the Miss Utah County Scholarship Pageant one August evening (and being voted, by my fellow contestants as "Miss Congeniality"), two of my fellow contestants exclaimed "Have you ever met Natalie Johnson? You are both so passionate about [fighting] cancer. You two are so similar; you're practically twin sisters […] Both of you would hit it off famously!" I had seen Natalie compete at Miss Utah two years prior and remembered her as an abundantly talented, poised, sophisticated, well-spoken, intelligent, and impressive woman who would be Miss Utah someday. In actual fact, I had seriously considered contacting her, on more than one occasion, to inquire about collaborating on different cancer education projects at the respective universities we attended. Alas, conflicting schedules provided it so that we never had an opportunity to officially meet face-to-face. That is, until Natalie was crowned Miss Utah the following year. It was June 15, 2002 and my life would forever be changed. My dedication to the cancer community would deepen; my love for service would increase tenfold and I would come to embrace my life's mission as a cancer crusader. And what began as a desire support the current Miss Utah and her platform grew into a profound respect for a remarkable human being, and, from there, into a genuine friendship. Indeed, I found a kindred spirit; my spirit twin. Suddenly, I had found a tiny silver lining in losing my mother to breast cancer—there was Natalie and, in turn, a birth of hope. In fighting skin cancer—the most preventable of all cancers—I found a sense of purpose. So, armed with hope and love, I, for the first time, really took up the crusade.

The first step in demonstrating my commitment to teaching other young adults about skin cancer prevention was for me to set the example; to practice what I preach. Though, initially motivated by a friend, I realized that my body is a gift. My body is sacred and therefore I must take of it. After all, if I am not taking care of myself, how can I possibly expect to take of others, especially my friends as well as the skin cancer community?

I researched dermatologists and found that several of the most well-respected melanoma skin cancer researchers were at Huntsman Cancer Institute in Salt Lake City, Utah—a mere three hour bus/train ride away from Provo, Utah. Needless to say, choosing a dermatologist who was right for me had little to do with the fact that I was a college senior with a limited income and without health insurance. At this point, I simply wanted to establish a relationship with a board-certified dermatologist that I truly connected with on a professional and interpersonal level. Perhaps, because I am a woman and we women tend to seek meaningful relationships that enrich and enhance our lives, the importance of choosing a dermatologist, of good reputation, with whom honest two-way communication is paramount, may seem "only natural." Nonetheless, I tell everyone else that I come in contact with that choosing a dermatologist ought to be based on variety of criteria which include personality and communicability, in addition to the fact that the dermatologist is in good standing with the American Academy of Dermatology and, hence, has received specialized training in skin cancer. When challenged by my first set of students who were being trained as peer skin cancer educators, I invited six well-respected dermatologist from across the United States to be guests on my weekly talk show to field questions and to share insights about key factors in establishing and maintaining effective, mutually-beneficial relationships with their dermatologist. All of them were in agreement. Good communication is vital for both doctor and patient, especially when preventing, detecting, diagnosing, and treating skin cancers. Dr. Hayes B. Gladstone, director of dermatologic surgery at Stanford University Medical Center in California, puts it this way:

> "Usually, if you have a friend or relative [who can refer you to their dermatologist] that is a good starting point. Web-sites, generally, provide good information about how good of a dermatologist a dermatologist is. Staff at a dermatologist's office should be polite and friendly. That is a good indication, too. If their staff is short or curt, that's not really a good sign."

Dr. Gladstone continues, "Do not go with a dermatologist that isn't a member of the American Academy of Dermatology. The AAD makes sure they get continually re-certified and trained. Most dermatologists are board certified." Moreover, I would emphasize a point that was addressed often throughout the nine months of interview dermatologists, patients, and survivors; a point that is best summed up by one single line that was uttered by Dr. Glen M. Bowen, the co-director of the Multi-disciplinary Melanoma Research Clinic at Huntsman Cancer Institute, on March 4, 2006: "Ultimately, any relationship enriches our lives, empowers patients, and enables doctors, which blesses all who actively participate in that relationship."

I could not have said it any better nor agree more.

Understanding both the role of a dermatologist and your role as the patient

First and foremost, it is essential that you recognize your individual responsibility as the patient and that you possess just as much responsibility in reducing your risk for a future skin cancer diagnosis. With that, never be afraid of opening your mouth. Ask questions and communicate, openly and honestly, with your dermatologist. True, the dermatologist has a profound responsibility in providing you with the best care possible but you can assist each other if you develop a sound understanding of both your role as patient and the dermatologist's role as the caregiver. This requires that you be a proactive participant and start this relationship on the right foot. Honestly, for someone who rarely scrambles for words to say and rarely fears open discussion, I was reluctant, if not intimidated, by the prospect of having to take off my clothes for that first initial full-body skin exam. Ultimately, I crippled myself by remaining silent, simply nodding my head and going through the motions. What a disservice I had done to both myself and to my dermatologist by not asking questions! It was unfortunate that, during my first visit, that I failed to seek clarification, voice my concerns, or even take notes to remind myself of the recommendations and suggestions that were given by the dermatologist. Certainly, I would have profited by having been adequately prepared. Knowing a few medical terms related to skin cancer, my dermatologist's education and professional history, and being aware that every inch of my body would be thoroughly examined, was not sufficient preparation. I needed to be armed with the tools to become my own best advocate; I needed to open my mouth. Often times we are taught to trust the experts and trust them we should. Yet, we must first trust ourselves and our ability to "know our body" by voicing any and all concerns. They matter how seemingly trivial they may be to us, because our dermatologist—if we have chosen the right one—wants to hear these concerns. They want to equip us with answers and tools to resolve those concerns. That said I have a checklist that I use to help myself prepare for my bi-annual visits to the dermatologist, and now use as a teaching aid when training college students to become peer educators on skin cancer. It is my so-called "In

Preparation for My First Visit Check List". (I urge you to customize it, a bit, based on your own personal skin cancer risk and medical history).

In Preparation for My First Visit Check List

- Medical records. Be sure to include information on family members if you have a family history of skin cancer. Though, skin cancer is largely caused by over-exposure to ultraviolet radiation from the sun, if you have had an immediate family member with skin cancer, particularly melanoma, you should make your dermatologist aware of it. Studies are underway at the Tom C. Mathews Jr. Familial Melanoma Research Clinic at Huntsman Cancer Institute about a p16 gene mutation and its link to melanoma so while 90-to-95% of skin carcinomas are attributed to ultraviolet radiation thus making it imperative that we properly protect ourselves from the sun (and avoid tanning beds), knowing our family history is also imperative.

- Notepad, Pen, and Tape Recorder. While my friends would say that I have a special knack for remembering what people say, trying to memorize every word my dermatologist says during an appointment is difficult, especially when I first meet with them. Visiting the dermatologist for the first time can be intimidating, if not nerve racking, so I recommend taking a tape recorder and notepad. This way, you can refer back to your notes, and play back the conversations that took place with your dermatologist. By doing this, you may have inadvertently missed a few key points amid sweating bullets during your first full-body skin exam. (A note on skin exams—don't sweat it. You don't have anything the dermatologist hasn't seen a thousand times before, so relax and bite the bullet).

- Your best friend, spouse, or another trusted confidant. I find that bringing someone I love with me when entering unfamiliar territory, helps put me at ease and allows me to simply "be myself." Suddenly, I forget to worry when I have someone I love and trust by my side holding my hand, so to speak, because I am comforted by a friendly, familiar face. Furthermore, having a companion there with you during your first initial visit to the dermatologist will definitely assist you with remembering specific recommendations the dermatologist made. Your companion may even ask questions you neglected to ask, thereby providing you with tools to establish a good relationship with your dermatologist.

- Medical dictionary. This will help familiarize you with specific dermatologic terms which, inevitably, will make for effective two-way communication between patient and dermatologist. I am reminded of being college. I would not dare go into class unprepared for fear the professor would ask me a question and discover that I had not sufficiently prepared. Besides, becoming familiar with key medical terms will lay down the foundation. It will provide a good framework thereby reducing any anxiety you may have in anticipation of that first visit with the dermatologist.

- A list of questions, particularly about your specific areas of concern (e.g., a suspicious mole or questionable "spot"). Unfortunately, many patients become crippled by a fear of asking questions, or asking "too many questions." To that, I say, yet again, *open your mouth!* If you do not articulate your feelings, thoughts, concerns, questions, even your fears, how can your dermatologist provide you with the answers you need? As with any relationship, trust must be present. In a relationship, each party must invest trust; to communicate openly and honestly is essential to building trust and in sustaining a viable relationship. So, swallow your fears, open your mouth, speak up, and really communicate with your dermatologist. Easier said than done, perhaps, but necessary. It could potentially save your life.

- Digital camera or digital photos. I add this to this list because I have numerous moles, many of which are dysplastic nevi (moles that have the potential of becoming melanoma). By taking pictures of my skin during monthly self skin exams, I can compare with the photos my dermatologist has on record thusly ensuring that neither one of us will miss any potential irregularities or changes in my skin. Remember, though your dermatologist is responsible for you, as the patient, you, too, are responsible for your own dermatologic health. For me, taking extra precautions and being proactive is about peace of mind. As Dr. Sancy A. Leachman, director of the Tom C. Mathews Jr. Familial Melanoma Research Clinic once told me: "An ounce of prevention is worth a pound of treatment." To which, I fully concur and often reiterate back to students. It is, indeed, better to be safe than sorry especially when dealing with cancer.

Facilitating effective communication between dermatologist and patient

Learning to communicate effectively with your dermatologist is a recurring theme addressed throughout this book, and that is completely intentional. The reason is not to be redundant; rather it is to emphasize the importance of how effective communication is a hugely significant component associated with skin cancer prevention, detection, and treatment, including surviving skin cancer. Honestly, for as well as I can carry a conversation, it was recently brought to my attention that, on occasion, I struggle with communicating effectively. It was my best friend Melissa that brought this to my attention, in her notoriously kind, gentle, loving yet straightforward and honest way, "Danielle, you have got to communicate your feelings *out loud*! Don't worry about what the other person might say or think, or how it may be perceived [...] don't let that prevent you from really saying what it is that worries you or concerns you. Give someone the chance to understand where you are coming from and to let them help you through your struggles. People care about you, so let them show it by helping you and serving you like you serve others so willingly and compassionately." Admittedly, I am quoting Melissa out-of-context. This statement was made in reference to a completely different conversation discussing a completely different issue; however, the crux is universally applicable. It is not necessarily what you said that is so important nor it is about how much you say; rather it is the quality of what you say. It is important to express yourself in an effective manner so that the other party can relate, empathize, understand, appreciate, and, in turn, appropriately respond. In sum, articulating your concerns about skin cancer ought to be more about carrying on a meaningful two-way conversation, as opposed to a reciting a listless series of scripted, standardized questions (though, I recommend taking a list of questions along with you to the dermatologist's office, as well as taking copious notes). Perhaps, if we saw our dermatologist as a human being who has our best interest in mind; a person who sincerely cares about our well-being and wants to help us, as opposed to a mere "figure head", per se, we would be less inhibited and less afraid to allow for that relationship to build and progress, thus allowing us to communicate effectively with our dermatologist.

Without fail, I will have at least one voice message or one email message from a woman inquiring about ways she can convince a man in her life—a husband, brother, father, or friend, to visit the dermatologist because she found "something suspicious on his skin."

Therefore, I have developed a few tricks of the trade to coax men into seeing the dermatologist. Bribery, coercion—I am not necessarily beneath exercising such methods when it involves the welfare of someone I love. That said here are a few suggestions to consider using on the reluctant man in your life and encourage him to regularly visit the dermatologist:

- Treat him to his favorite restaurant or to a romantic weekend. Perhaps, you can even agree to let him have full possession of the remote control for an entire week. (Personally, I have found that food is a secure way to a man's heart; however, other men are motivated by the prospect of uncensored access to sports television, et. al.).

- Guilt him into it. "If you love me, you would go to the dermatologist." Remind the man that he has people who care for and love him, as well as well as people who depend on him. If he refuses to take care of himself, he is not only letting himself down but others, as well.

- Recruit back up. Work with his closet buddies, co-workers, or even his boss. Recently, my boss and I ganged up on the vice president of our department. After realizing our genuine care and concern, he agreed to schedule an appointment with his dermatologist that very day. He did and he followed through on his promise by keeping the appointment he scheduled, because he wanted to "do it for his family." It is difficult not to surrender and comply when cornered, especially by those we care for and respect; by people who are genuinely and altruistically interested in our overall well-being.

- Make it a team effort. You can offer to examine his skin for him and, in turn, can perform the monthly self-skin exams for you.

- Reward him. When he comes home from his visit to the dermatologist, he may feel vulnerable. After all, a full-body skin exam is not the most pleasant experience. Reward him for his efforts. Depending on his preference, reward him with tickets to an upcoming sporting event or concert, and, of course, plenty of affection and praise.

- Tell him outright. Men avoid doctors because they hate to face their own mortality, or feel as though they aren't in control, so ladies help him out by telling him how much you love and care for him. Tell the man in your life, whether it be a husband, father, brother, or friend that you love him and his welfare is important to you and, as such, you would like to take them into see the dermatologist.

Understanding your melanoma risk

As mentioned previously, everyone is at risk for melanoma; however, others possess a higher risk for this deadly, yet preventable, disease. While, familial melanoma (melanoma among families) only accounts for less than 10% of all diagnosed cases of melanoma, revolutionary research about the genetics behind melanoma are underway at Huntsman Cancer Institute in Salt Lake City. Dr. Sancy A. Leachman, principle investigator at the Tom C. Mathews Jr. Familial Melanoma Research Clinic at HCI, is leading research on familial melanoma and, hence, is shedding light on this complex form of cancer to better understand an individual's likelihood for melanoma.

Several years ago, researchers at the University of Utah School of Medicine conducted a series of studies on families considered "high risk" for melanoma skin cancer. By analyzing their medical history, their genealogy, coupled with various blood and tissue samples, scientists and oncologists were able to isolate and identify a specific gene mutation called a p16. This gene, when mutated, increases one's likelihood for melanoma; however. According to Leachman, "though some cancer-causing gene mutations are passed down from one generation to another" the chief culprit behind the p16 gene mutation associated with melanoma occurs "when a person spends too much time in the sun [and] has one or more severe sunburns.

> "When p16 is not working properly, skin cells reproduce out of control, leading to melanoma. People who know they have an increased risk for skin cancer because of light hair or fair skin or other inherited factors, such as a gene mutation, should take the appropriate screening and prevention measures to help protect themselves from developing the disease."

In sum, over-exposure to ultraviolet radiation is considered the most conclusive factor in increasing an individual's likelihood for a future melanoma; however, if you have numerous dysplastic nevi (atypical moles) and/or have had an immediate family member suffer melanoma, you should consult your dermatologist and insist on regular screenings. You may want to also consider being a part research studies akin to those taking place at Huntsman Cancer Institute at the University of Utah.

Coping with a skin cancer diagnosis

As you cope with cancer and cancer treatment, you need to have honest, open discussions with your doctor. You should feel free to ask any question that is on your mind no matter how awkward it might seem. Nurses, social workers, and other members of the treatment team may also be able to answer many of your questions. Here is a list of questions you might want to ask your dermatologists:

- What type of skin cancer do I have?
- Can you explain the different types of skin cancer?
- Are there any specific signs or symptoms that I should be aware of or look for?
- Has my cancer spread beneath the skin? Has it spread to lymph nodes or other organs?
- What are my treatment options? What do you recommend? Why?
- Will I be okay if the cancer is just removed with no follow-up treatment?
- What are the risks or side effects that I should expect?
- Will a scar remain after treatment?
- What are the chances of my cancer coming back with the treatment options we have discussed?
- What should I do to be ready for treatment?
- What is my expected prognosis, based on my cancer as you view it?
- What are my chances of developing another skin cancer?
- Should I take special precautions to avoid sun exposure? What are the most important steps I can take to protect myself from the sun?
- Are any of my family members at risk for skin cancer? What should I tell them to do? Should I tell my children's pediatrician that I have been diagnosed with a skin cancer?

In addition to these sample questions, be sure to write down any additional questions you may have for the dermatologist. For instance, you might want more information about recovery times so that you can plan your work schedule. You may want to inquire about second opinions or about clinical trials for which you may qualify. Remember, you must be an active participant in the process. As Dr. Glen M. Bowen, director of the Multi-disciplinary Melanoma Research Clinic at Huntsman Cancer Institute puts it: "You have to take some responsibility as a patient. Me being a doctor, I've also been a patient, and I can't stress enough that you have to take some responsibility. This isn't like getting on a roller coaster and having the seatbelt clasped, and you just go along for the ride. You have to take some responsibility for what's going on [with your health]."

Treatment options and procedures

Fortunately, with continued advancements in melanoma research, a variety of treatments are available for melanoma. If you, or a loved one, should receive a diagnosis of melanoma, your oncologist will suggest a course of action based on the location, type and stage of a disease, your age, and your general health. Following is a list, provided by the American Academy of Dermatology, of treatment options for melanoma:

When the melanoma spreads to one area:

The primary treatment for melanoma that spreads to one site is surgical removal of the melanoma. In some cases, surgical removal may not be feasible or may not be able to remove all of the cancer. In these cases, stage IV melanoma that has spread to one area may be treated with:

- Chemotherapy—Chemotherapy is the use of cancer-fighting medications to stop the growth of malignant cells. In stage IV melanoma, systemic (affects the entire body) chemotherapy is used. One medication that may be used is dacarbazine (DTIC), which is approved by the U.S. Food and Drug Administration (FDA) for treating melanoma. DTIC is given intravenously for 1 to 10 days. The dosing schedule depends on the patient's condition and ability to tolerate side effects, which may include nausea, vomiting, pain at the injection site, and fatigue. DTIC often is used in combination with another cancer medication(s) as research shows this can increase effectiveness. Another chemotherapeutic medication used to treat stage IV melanoma is temozolomide, which may be administered alone or with another medication.

- Close observation—This option involves delaying treatment for up to three months and repeating scans and other medical tests to see if the melanoma continues to spread. If the melanoma does not spread and it is believed that surgery will remove the melanoma, surgery is performed. Sometimes surgery cures the cancer.

- Immunotherapy—Immunotherapy uses medication to stimulate or enhance the patient's immune responses in order to fight established cancer. In stage IV, the systemic medication, interluekin-2 (IL-2), may be used.

- Palliative care—The purpose of this type of therapy is to relieve symptoms and improve a patient's quality of life, not treat the cancer. Patients in all stages may receive palliative care. In advanced stages, palliative care can help control the symptoms and pain. Radiation therapy is a type of palliative care used in stage IV melanoma to relieve symptoms and ease pain.

Adjuvant therapy—After surgery, one of the following adjuvant therapies is usually recommended if it appears that the cancer has been removed:

- Clinical trial—A clinical trial may be recommended when it is believed the treatment being studied can benefit the patient. If this is a consideration, the patient should discuss the potential risks and benefits with a doctor who is treating the patient for melanoma. The decision of whether or not to enroll in a clinical trial rests completely with the patient.

- Close observation—The patient does not undergo further treatment but returns for frequent physical examinations and/or diagnostic tests that can detect cancer.

- Interferon injections—To help boost the patient's immune system, injections of interferon-alpha may be given. Interferons are naturally produced by the body's immune system. However, as a medication, interferon-alpha can produce undesirable side effects, including aches, chills, fever, and extreme fatigue. Interferon-alpha also can affect the heart and liver, so it should only be administered by a physician who is experienced in using this treatment to minimize side effects and increase effectiveness.

If all of the cancer cannot be removed, then systemic (affects the entire body) treatment with chemotherapy (cancer-fighting medications) or immunotherapy (medication used to boost the patient's immune system) may be recommended.

When the melanoma spreads to multiple areas: Treatment options include:

- Chemotherapy—Chemotherapy is the use of cancer-fighting medications to stop the growth of malignant cells. Systemic (affects the entire body) chemotherapy with the medication dacarbazine (DTIC) may be used. DTIC is FDA-approved for treating melanoma. DTIC often is used in combination with other cancer medication(s) as research shows this can increase effectiveness. Another chemotherapeutic medication used to treat stage IV melanoma is temozolomide, which also may be administered alone or with other medication(s).

- Clinical trial—This is the method most often used to treat a patient with stage IV melanoma when the cancer spreads to multiple areas.

- Immunotherapy—Immunotherapy uses medication to stimulate or enhance the patient's immune responses in order to fight established cancer. In stage IV, the systemic medication, interluekin-2 (IL-2), may be used.

- Palliative care—The purpose of this therapy is to relieve symptoms and improve a patient's quality of life, not treat the cancer. Patients in all stages may receive palliative care. In advanced stages, palliative care can help control the symptoms and pain. Radiation therapy is used for this purpose in stage IV.

Recurrence: If melanoma recurs (returns), the patient may receive:

- Surgery to remove the tumor.

- Treatment via clinical trial. This may involve chemotherapy (medication used to kill cancer cells or stop them from dividing) or immunotherapy (treatment to help the patient's immune system fight the cancer).

- Palliative care. When melanoma recurs, immunotherapy may be used to ease symptoms and improve the quality of life instead of treat the cancer. Easing discomfort rather than treating the condition is known as palliative care. Radiation therapy also may provide palliative care when melanoma recurs.

With that, let it be said that follow-up is an essential part to treatment, because melanoma can return and spread. After treatment, patients are taught how to carefully and properly examine their own skin and lymph nodes for melanoma. Patients are also instructed on how to detect warning signs and symptoms, such as cough and chest pain, which may indicate that melanoma, has spread to other parts of the body. It is important to perform these examinations as instructed to be able to recognize signs and symptoms. If any changes occur, immediately report any changes to your doctor. Studies show that the majority of metastases (spreads) and recurrences (melanoma returns) are discovered by the patient or a family member. One study, according to the American Academy of Dermatology, found that self-examination often results in earlier detection of melanoma when it is still surgically curable. Equally important, patients should keep all appointments for follow-up visits. Research shows that numerous metastases, local recurrences, and second primary melanomas are detected by a physician during routine examinations. Case-in-point:

It was April 2, 2006. I was in the shower and, noticing out of the corner of my eye, the self-skin examination card I had hanging from the shower head (which neighbors my self-breast examination card), I was reminded that it was probably about time to perform my monthly self-skin exam. While doing this, I had noticed that a mole, located in the bend of my left knee, appeared larger. This particular mole has never been one that I worried about, unlike the many dysplastic nevi (abnormal moles) located on my back; however, this one, on this day, appeared as though it were growing laterally across my skin. After wrestling with this concern for several days, I eventually scheduled an appointment with the dermatologist. When I called and said, "I think I have a mole that is growing", the response it yielded was "Get in here right NOW!" Thankfully, the mole was and still is benign. It was not, in fact, growing laterally across my skin, as it had appeared. While my concern was unwarranted, the peace of mind squelched my fears and reminded me of the value, and the importance, of performing my monthly self-skin exams. If I ever should have a mole that is, indeed, changing, I will be able to, more than likely, catch it before it becomes malignant.

In sum, always consult the qualified advice of a board-certified dermatologist-oncologist. I also urge you to insist on being made aware of all available and viable options of treatment (as well as the side effects, success rates, and other related consequences) when facing a melanoma diagnosis.

The basics of preventing the most preventable cancer

In previous sections, skin cancer has been defined as a term designating the uncontrolled growth of immature cells in the skin; however, despite a heightened risk due to external environmental factors, proven effective preventive measures exist to facilitate a combative stance against skin cancer. These proven prevention measures include proper use of sunscreens with a SPF of at least 15, wearing wide-brimmed hats and UV protective clothing, avoiding direct sunlight—year round—between the peak hours of 10:00 a.m. and 4:00 p.m., and performing monthly skin exams. Challenging skin cancer prevention education efforts, however, is the disparity in awareness and action stimulated as a by-product of popular culture. A recent study demonstrates this disparity.

The American Academy of Dermatology learned, through a May 2005 survey of 505 teenagers between the ages of 12-and-17, that 66% of them were [are] aware that ultraviolet radiation from the sun is a large, if not primary, culprit behind one's risk for getting skin cancer, but more then 47% of them still reported that did not discourage nor deter them from seeking a tan. Furthermore, over 80% of the teens surveyed reported having knowledge of the fact that sustaining sunburn as a child dramatically increases an individual's likelihood of having a future skin cancer as an adult; however, 60% of them admitted to suffering sunburns last summer. In other words, 52% of the adolescents surveyed by the AAD reported that "they are not too careful or not at all careful to protect their skin from sun exposure," according to Jennifer Allyn, senior public relations specialist for the AAD. Dr. Saraiya of the CDC puts it this way: "While knowledge of the risk of sun exposure and the use of sunscreens and other forms of sun protection have improved over the past two decades, a gap still exists between knowledge and behavior."

Despite this disparity, one ought to consider how being taught at an early age, we, as adults, "automatically" brush our teeth, take a shower, put on clean clothes, and therefore perform the other rituals that comprise our daily morning routine. Proper maintenance and hygiene was learned, from an early age, and became habit through repeated performances of those learned practices. Apply the same principle when properly applying an ample amount of SPF 15 sunscreen, slapping on a wide-brimmed hat, and sporting the hottest pair of UV protective shades before heading outdoors each day. Albeit, there are catchy slogans and acronyms to jog your memory about practicing proper prevention such as: "It's As Easy Your ABC's" used by the Utah Cancer Action Network: A = Avoid the sun in the middle of the day; B = Block the sun by applying sunscreen; C = Continuously take sun safety precautions. Perhaps, more well-known and used (especially among those in the field of dermatology) is the slogan borrowed from our friends in Australia: "Slip, Slap, Slop!" We, at The Cancer Crusaders Organization, along with the nationally-ranked Utah Valley State dance team, turned the "Slip, Slap, Slop!" slogan into a cheer, in honor of skin cancer survivor, Robin Lawrence (read about her incredible story in Part IV).

Slip. Slip on a long-sleeved shirt/Slap. Slap on a wide-brimmed hat/Slop. Slop on a SPF 15 sunscreen everyday/Slip, Slap, Slop! Slip, Slap, Slop—that's the SunSavvy® way!

Whether it be a fancy tune, a silly cheer, or any other cleverly packaged pneumonic device to get you into the groove, the basics of skin cancer prevention are only effective if properly practiced on a regular basis—every day, year-round, for life.

Choosing a sunscreen and maximizing its efficacy

Consider this: What if you could be armed with an invisible force field that would protect you and your loved ones form any unseen dangers and harm? Sounds good, right? To have a secure way of ensuring you and your loved ones are safe every day, would definitely make your life easier And what if I told you that your search for this invisible bulletproof vest has been right under your nose—that you can get it at your favorite dermatologist's office? That lifesaving product is none other than sunscreen.

Truth be told, sunscreen, when used properly, works much akin to a coat of armor. It is akin to an invisible bulletproof vest that contains organic molecules that absorb, scatter and reflect ultraviolet radiation, thus protecting you and your family members from a silent killer called the sun. Over-exposure to UV rays means a significantly heightened risk for skin cancer, which is most the commonly diagnosed cancer in the world (and, yet, it is also the most preventable). As you will recall, from Part I, every hour another American succumbs to melanoma skin cancer, according to the AAD.

Two decades ago, sunscreen was relatively unheard of, whereas today it has become almost common jargon. Increased awareness of skin cancer and the importance of sunscreen, even sun protective clothing have, in ways, only further confused us and perhaps even caused us to ignore the warnings. Have you ever wondered why there have been occasions when you slapped on a pound of SPF 45 before hitting the beach or the slopes only return home burnt to a crisp? The problem is, we are told to use sunscreen but we are not instructed on how to properly apply it so as to maximize its efficacy.

Unlike a bulletproof vest, however, sunscreen must be re-applied in order for it to properly provide protection from ultraviolet radiation. Consider the 30-20-2 rule: Apply an SPF 15 sunscreen on at least 30-minutes prior to going outdoors—even on cloudy days—and, then, reapply it within the first 20-minutes of being outside, and then apply consistently in two hour intervals. (For children under 18, sunscreen must be applied every hour). The reason sunscreen works this way is based on the mechanics of our skin.

Our skin works much like a sponge does. The top layer, the epidermis, absorbs sunscreen, forming a protective layer atop the skin that "blocks" UV rays from reaching the melanocytes that lie deep within the skin. Yet, our skin, like sponge, reaches a saturation point. This saturation point occurs after approximately two hours, thus leaving you unprotected from ultraviolet radiation exposure and causing sunburn and other skin-related damage. Hence, it is imperative that a broad-spectrum sunscreen be reapplied in order to maximize its protective powers.

Alas, not all sunscreen products out on the market today work proficiently. To deliver an optimum level of protection, a sunscreen must have sufficient quantities of essential ingredients. In other words, when choosing the best sunscreen product for you and your family, take a look at the bottle; make sure it contains proven effective agents such as zinc oxide and titanium dioxide. Also, make sure the product is a broad-spectrum formula, meaning that it blocks both UV-B and UV-A rays. If the sunscreen is not broad-spectrum, do not buy it. You are not being sufficiently protected or "covered" by a non-broad-spectrum sunscreen,

The significance of a broad-spectrum sunscreen cannot be over-emphasized. UV-B and UV-A rays have varied affects on your skin, your immune system, and your body as a whole. UV-B irradiation disrupts the melanocytes, causing them to release the "redness" known as sunburn. Any change in the color of your skin as a result of over-exposure to ultraviolet radiation is damage to your skin, even if your skin tends to tan as opposed to burn. Any change in your skin pigmentation is your melanocytes way of telling you that normal, healthy cells have been severely disrupted and, thus, they are trying to compensate for the damage they have sustained (but, keep in mind that photo damage from ultraviolet radiation is un-repairable). On the other hand, damage to your skin caused by UV-A irradiation is far more serious. UV-A rays are especially harmful as they penetrate deep beneath your epidermis, into the layer underneath known as the dermis. Typically, the immediate affects of UV-A rays are not visible, but they are the chief culprit behind photo-aging and wrinkling. Have you ever left a basketball outside in the hot summer sun for a lengthy period of time? Then, when you went to retrieve the ball, you almost immediately notice that the elasticity of the ball has weakened. The ball feels melted and never quite bounces back. This is exactly what happens to your skin as a result of prolonged UV-A exposure. Both UV-B and UV-A rays have cumulative affects and coupled together can lead to skin cancer. Ultraviolet radiation is a known carcinogen that adversely damaging affects on a variety of biological systems.

With that said, make sure you understand "SPF" when purchasing a brand of sunscreen, and do not be mislead by brands that only claim to deliver a high level of protection. To begin with, SPF stands for sun protection factor (or "sunburn protection factor"). The way SPF works can be best described by the following example: A SPF 20 sunscreen is only allowing five out of every 100 UV protons to reach your skin. In other words, it is protecting you from an estimated 95% of UV rays. Therefore it is strongly recommended that a SPF 15 sunscreen be used year-round, even on cloudy days. Yet, if you are planning a long, leisurely day at the lake or even a marathon day on the ski slopes, you will want to opt for a SPF 30 and be sure to re-apply every hour to prevent a painful reminder of your day of recreation. It is noteworthy to mention that, according to the American Cancer Society, 60% of Americans suffered [at least] one severe "blistering" sunburn in 2004 as a result of improper sunscreen application and use. Could this lack of proper sun safety be contributing to the ever-increasing skin cancer incidence? How many skin cancers could be avoided if we were to only properly use a SPF 15 broad-spectrum sunscreen? Certainly the world's most common cancer can be prevented if we are more proactive about properly protecting ourselves with adequate sunscreen. Would a warrior leave to face a battle without being adequately armed with protection or equipped with the proper weapons to defend themselves from the enemy at-hand? Therefore, we must be sure to properly and regularly apply sunscreen to our skin. After all, it is the closest to a bulletproof vest we have against a growing epidemic known as skin cancer.

As always, skin cancer educators trust the authority on the matter—the American Academy of Dermatology. The AAD and Del-Ray Dermatologicals, the manufacturers Blue Lizard Australian Sunscreen, have provided a comprehensive, yet easy-to-understand list of facts about sunscreens, (which we have edited, modified, and added to, for the purposes of this book):
Fact about Sunscreen:

- **What is sunscreen?** Sunscreens are products that protect the skin from damage caused by ultraviolet radiation (UVR). They do this by using: organic chemicals that absorb light and dissipate it as heat; inorganic filters (blockers) that sit on the surface of the skin and act as physical barriers; or a combination of both.

- **Who needs to use sunscreen?** In a word: Everyone. The American Academy of Dermatology suggests that, regardless of skin type, a broad-spectrum (protects against UV-A and UV-B rays) sunscreen with a sun protection factor (SPF) of at least 15 should be used year-round.

- **When should sunscreen be used?** Sunscreens should be used every day, year-round if you are going to be in the sun for more than 20 minutes. They can be applied under makeup and cosmetics. A variety of cosmetic and skin care products available today contain sunscreens for daily use because sun protection is the principal means of preventing premature aging and skin cancer; however, it is recommend that sunscreen be applied, in addition, to this since, after about two hours, the sunscreen has been absorbed by the skin. Since the sun is responsible for the production of vitamin D in the skin, there is debate whether or not sunscreen users ought to be concerned about their vitamin D levels. The AAD strongly discourages using the sun as a means of vitamin D production, as it places one at higher risk for skin cancer. As such, people should take a multivitamin or drink vitamin D fortified milk. The reflective powers of the sun are great—17% on sand and 80% percent on snow. Do not reserve the use of these products only for sunny summer days. Even on a cloudy day, 80% of the ultraviolet rays pass through the clouds, therefore it is imperative that sunscreen be properly applied on a regular, daily basis.

- **How much sunscreen should be used and how often should it be applied?** Sunscreens should be applied to dry skin approximately 30 minutes prior to going outdoors. When applying sunscreen, pay particular attention to the face, ears, hands and arms, and coat the skin liberally. One ounce (enough to fill a shot glass), is considered the amount needed to cover the exposed areas of the body properly. Be careful to cover exposed areas completely—a missed spot could mean a painful sunburn. Do not forget that lips get sunburned too, so apply a lip balm that contains sunscreen, preferably with an SPF 15 or higher. Sunscreens should be re-applied every two hours or after swimming or perspiring heavily. Even so-called water resistant sunscreens may lose their effectiveness after 80 minutes in the water. Sunscreens rub off as well as wash off, so if you have towel-dried, reapply waterproof sunscreen for continued protection. Do not forget that sun exposure occurs all the time, even when you are on a short walk on a cloudy day.

- **What type of sunscreen should I use, and what ingredients should I look for?** There are so many types of sunscreen that selecting the right one can be quite confusing. Sunscreens are available in many forms including ointments, creams, gels, lotions and wax sticks. The type of sunscreen you choose is a matter of personal choice. Ideally, sunscreens should be water resistant, so they cannot be easily removed by sweating or swimming, and should have an SPF 15 or higher that provides broad-spectrum coverage against all ultraviolet light wavelengths. Ingredients which provide broad-spectrum protection include benzophenones (oxybenzone), cinnamates (octylmethyl cinnamate and cinoxate), sulisobenzone, salicylates, titanium dioxide, zinc oxide, and avobenzone (Parsol 1789®). (Note: According to Australian standards, which are considered the strictest in the world, the best protection ingredients include a minimum 5% of titanium dioxide and a minimum 5% of titanium dioxide).

- **Can I use the sunscreen I bought last summer, or do I need to purchase a new bottle each year? Does it lose its strength and potency?** Unless indicated by an expiration date, the Food and Drug Administration (FDA) requires that all sunscreens be stable and at their original strength for at least three years. While you can use the sunscreen that you bought last summer, keep in mind that if you are using the appropriate amount, a bottle of sunscreen should not last you very long. Approximately one ounce of sunscreen, enough to fill a shot glass, is considered the amount needed to cover the exposed areas of the body properly.

- **What is the difference between UV-A and UV-B ultraviolet light wavelengths and will a sunscreen protect me from both?** Sunlight consists of two types of harmful rays—UV-A rays and UV-B rays. The UV-B rays are the sun's burning rays (which are blocked by window glass) and are the primary cause of sunburn and skin cancer. UV-A rays (which pass through window glass) penetrate deeper into the dermis, or base layer of the skin. They also contribute to sunburns and skin cancer. Both UV-A and UV-B rays can cause suppression of the immune system which helps to protect you against the development and spread of skin cancer. Since PABA and PABA esters only protect against UV-B light, check for a broad-spectrum sunscreen that also screens UV-A rays. Ingredients like benzophenones, oxybenzone, sulisobenzone, titanium dioxide, zinc oxide, and avobenzone (Parsol 1789), extend the coverage beyond the UV-B range and into the UV-A range, helping to make sunscreens broad-spectrum.

- **What is an SPF?** SPF stands for sun protection factor. Sunscreens are rated or classified, by the strength of their SPF. The SPF numbers on the packaging can range from as low as two to greater than 50. These numbers refer to the sunscreens ability to deflect ultraviolet radiation. The sunscreen SPF rating is calculated by comparing the amount of time needed to produce a sunburn on sunscreen protected skin to the amount of time needed to cause a sunburn on unprotected skin. For example, if a sunscreen is rated SPF 2 and a fair-skinned person who would normally turn red after 10 minutes of exposure in the sun uses that, it would take

20 minutes of exposure for the skin to turn red. A sunscreen with an SPF of 15 would allow that person to multiply that initial burning time by 15, which means it would take 15 times longer to burn, or 150 minutes. Let it be reiterated that dermatologists strongly recommend using a broad-spectrum sunscreen with a minimum SPF 15 year-round for all skin types. (Note: Molecularly there exists no formula stronger than SPF 30, so be weary of sunscreens claiming to be higher than an SPF 30, as they are likely a marketing ploy).

- **Does SPF 30 have twice as much sun protection as SPF 15?** SPF protection does not actually increase proportionately with a designated SPF number. In higher SPFs, such as an SPF of 30, 97% of sunburning rays are deflected, while an SPF of 15 indicates 93% deflection and an SPF of 2 equals 50-percent deflection. Research suggests that high SPF sunscreens are an appropriate choice for very sun sensitive individuals. One study determined that skin protected by an SPF 15 sunscreen and then exposed to 15 times the minimum dose of sunlight normally required to cause redness produced 2.5 times the number of sunburn cells seen in SPF 30 protected skin with the same dose of sunlight. These results suggest that prevention of redness does not necessarily mean prevention of all sun-induced damage. More research is currently underway on the protective effects of sunscreens on different skin types.

- **What kind of protection do sunscreens provide?** SPF 30 sunscreens filter 97% of UV-B rays. In Australia, broad-spectrum sunscreens must protect against 90% or more of UV-A rays. In the United States, there is no approved evaluation of UV-A protection, therefore a broad-spectrum label is open to interpretation. Consumers should be educated on the ingredients that provide UV-A protection. Products that contain 6% or more zinc oxide provide excellent UV-A protection.

- **Does the SPF tell how well a sunscreen protects against UV-A or UV-B rays?** The SPF number on sunscreens only reflects the ability of the sunscreen screen for UV-B rays. At present, there is not a FDA-approved rating system that identifies UV-A protection. Scientists are working to create a standardized testing system to measure UV-A protection.

- **What is the difference between a sunscreen and a sunblock?** Since sunscreens can now either chemically absorb ultraviolet radiation, or deflect them, the term sunblock is no longer used. It is important to find a sunscreen that offers both UV-A and UV-B (broad spectrum) protection and includes ingredients zinc oxide and titanium dioxide.

- **Is sunscreen application all I need to do to protect myself from the sun?** Because over-exposure to ultraviolet light is the primary cause of melanoma, dermatologists recommend the following precautions:

  - Avoid the "peak" hours of 10:00 a.m. -and- 4:00 p.m. when ultraviolet rays from the sun are strongest.

  - Seek shade whenever possible. *No shadow, seek the shade!* If your shadow is shorter than you are, the damaging rays of the sun are at their strongest and you are most likely to sunburn.

  - Apply a broad-spectrum sunscreen with a sun protection factor (SPF) 15 or higher, apply 30 minutes before going outdoors and re-apply every two hours. (Re-apply sunscreen every hour if you are planning to be outdoors for a considerable amount of time especially when playing, gardening, swimming or doing any other outdoor activities). Sunscreens should not be used to increase the time spent in intense sunlight nor replace protective clothing.

  - Wear protective clothing, including a wide-brimmed hat, UV protective wrap-around sunglasses, a long-sleeved shirt and pants during prolonged periods of sun exposure.

- **Is there a safe way to tan?** *There is NO safe way to tan!* A tan indicates skin damage and injury. Tanning occurs when the ultraviolet rays penetrate the dermis (the inner layer of the skin), causing the skin to produce more melanin (pigmentation) as a response to the injury. Chronic exposure to ultraviolet radiation results in a change in the texture of the skin causing wrinkling and age spots. Thus, tanning to improve appearance is ultimately self-defeating. Every time you tan, you accumulate damage to the skin. This damage, in addition to accelerating the aging process, also increases your risk for all types of skin cancer, including melanoma. A number of studies have confirmed that repeated sunburns and tans substantially increase the risk for melanoma. This is especially true for childhood sunburns because there is more time and opportunity for subsequent sun damage to lead to melanoma.

- **Are tanning booths a safer way to tan?** In spite of claims that tanning booths offer "safe" tanning, artificial radiation carries all the risks of natural sunlight. Hence, *there is no such thing as a safe tan.* Period. Tanning booths emit UV-A radiation, which poses both short and long-term risks to the skin, including cataracts (eye damage), sunburns, skin cancer and premature aging. In addition, there can be damage to the body's immune system and reactions to certain fragrances, lotions, moisturizers and medications. Many tanning salons are unregulated, allowing customers (especially those whose skin is incapable of tanning) access to tanning beds without supervision or eye protection. The American Academy of Dermatology supports local and/or statewide indoor tanning legislation that bans minors from using tanning devices. In addition, this legislation usually requires that warning signs be prominently displayed in tanning salons and list the hazards of such exposure, among other possible regulatory provisions.

- **How much sunscreen should I apply to my skin each day to make sure I am covered?** Considered the authority on the proper use of sunscreens, Dr. Elma Baron of Case Western Reserve University in Cleveland, Ohio, strongly recommends using an ounce of sunscreen (or the equivalent to the amount that would fit into the palm of your hand). With that, it is imperative to remember to apply sunscreen on every inch of your body that is [potentially] exposed to UV rays. Places such as your ears, behind your neck, your back, the backs of your calves, your toes, are all places that are commonly neglected. If you have trouble reaching certain parts of your body, get your spouse or your best friend to help you apply sunscreen. Make it a team effort to protect each other from the sun.

- **Which sunscreens on the market today are best for my budget?** Dr. Sancy A. Leachman, deputy director and principle investigator at the Tom C. Mathews Jr. Familial Melanoma Research Clinic at Huntsman Cancer Institute in Salt Lake City, Utah, has put together an exhaustive and accurate spreadsheet that lists every sunscreen product imaginable; lists them by the amount of essential protective ingredients each products incorporates in its sunscreen formula, the level of SPF it provides, and how much the product cost per ounce in comparison to its competitors. To reference Dr. Leachman's An Ounce of Prevention sunscreen spreadsheet, please send an email to **info@cancercrusaders.org**

- **Are men or women better about regular sunscreen usage?** It is interesting to note results from a survey conducted by the American Academy of Dermatology in May 2005. Through this survey, the AAD learned that teenage boys are the least likely of all Americans to use sunscreen. Only 32% of teenage boys aged 15-to-17 reported taking regular precautions against over-exposure to ultraviolet rays. Similarly, the U.S. Surgeon General Richard H. Carmona, M.D., MPH, reports a survey conducted by the Sun Safety Alliance, reflects that sunscreen usage among Americans in their 20s and 30s is decreasing; from 72% last year to less than 60%

today. In general, though, middle-aged women are better about sunscreen usage—85%, on average, reported knowing "the dangers of overexposure to the sun and believe skin cancer is a serious issue." Yet, what is perplexing to us is that if the vast majority of American adults claim to know about the dangers of skin cancer, than why did over 60% of Americans sustained sunburn last year? It is bewildering that, despite that people are aware of the fact that nearly 90% of skin cancers are caused by over-exposure to ultraviolet radiation (and that the main source of those UV rays are from the sun), there is still a lack of proactive preventative behaviors being practiced. Dr. Carmona reports that one in 1 in 3 Americans "simply forget" to apply sunscreen. To us, forgetfulness is not an excuse. Properly using sunscreen needs to become a part of our daily routine in order for it to become a lifelong habit. And as with any other habit, it takes constant repetition before it becomes a behavior.

- **What are some clever ways for me to remember to use my sunscreen and to bring it with me as I leave the house each morning?** We, at The Cancer Crusaders Organization, have a few ideas about how to incorporate a regular practice of proper sunscreen usage so as to foster a permanent lifelong habit. To mention a few: 1) Consider placing a bottle of sunscreen in your make-up bag or by your bathroom sink (right next to your toothbrush and toothpaste); 2) Consider getting a bottle of sunscreen that has a key ring on it and fastening it to your house and/or car keys; 3) Put post-it notes on your mirrors or on the front door that read: *STOP! Put on your sunscreen right NOW!* Do this until it becomes so natural that you do not even have to even "think" about it because you are doing it all the time anyway; it becomes automatic; it becomes a habit. You can also ask your spouse, your room-mates, your friends, or your loved ones, to give you friendly reminders. (Be aware that these friendly reminders may seem annoying, but you asked for it).

- **Does sunscreen, especially sunscreen usage as a child, really reduce your risk for skin cancer?** If you recall, the AAD reports 80% of our lifetime sun damage is sustained during our first 18 years of life, therefore making a habit of daily, year-round sunscreen usage beginning in childhood is good common sense. And, yes, sunscreen use in children can lower one's risk for skin cancer in the future. "Sunscreen has always been an important part of an overall sun safety regime to protect the number of sunburns, especially for children," reports dermatologist Jason K. Rivers of the University of British Columbia Department of Medicine. Dr. Rivers conducted a study of 309 Caucasian children ages six-to-10, who were monitored for three years. "[…] children with sunscreen develop less nevi (moles), it is of some significance."

- **Does sunscreen cause a vitamin D deficiency?** As mentioned previously, our bodies need vitamin D because it helps with the production of calcium and phosphorus—two minerals necessary for the building and maintenance of strong, healthy bones. Alas, the sun, or any other form of ultraviolet radiation, is not a viable method of getting your daily vitamin D. We have mentioned how ultraviolet radiation damages our skin and places us at a significantly higher risk for skin cancer, so to justify the use of indoor tanning beds or "laying out" on the beach as a means of getting vitamin D is not only dangerous, but unnecessary. Americans fortify a majority of their grocery products with vitamin D. Consider milk, for example. If we have a bowl of cereal every day you would get sufficient vitamin D.

Key points about sunscreens:

- No sunscreen is "waterproof" or "sweatproof". Sunscreen should always be applied to dry skin. All sunscreens start to come off during activity; it is important that sunscreen be reapplied after towel drying. Products labeled as "waterproof" in the United States have completed an 80-minute still-water bath test. Products labeled as "very water resistant" in Australia retain their SPF after 240 minutes in moving water. Australia does not allow the use of "waterproof" or "sweat-proof", and the Food and Drug Administration asked for voluntary removal.

- No sunscreen provides "all-day protection". As stated, chemical absorbers work by absorbing light, but they can be photo unstable. For example, avobenzone loses 36% of its effectiveness within the first 15 minutes of sun exposure. Inorganic filters (zinc oxide and titanium dioxide) adhere to the skin but can be removed during towel drying. Australia does not allow the use of labels that read "all-day protection." Once again, the FDA has asked for voluntary removal of this label claim.

- High SPF sunscreens do not necessarily offer broader or better protection. SPF only indicates the amount of UV-B protection a product provides and does not indicate how much if any UV-A protection is provided. The consumer needs to understand that the specific formulation of the sunscreen determines the amount of protection provided. Zinc Oxide products (6% or higher) provide very photostable UV-B and UV-A protection. High SPF products (e.g. SPF 45, 55, 60) typically contain high levels of organic chemicals that can increase the potential for irritation and absorption, especially in children. Higher is not always better, which is why Australia limits SPF label claims to 30.

- No sunscreen offers complete protection against the sun. Therefore products using the term "sunblock" are a misnomer as they do allow some ultraviolet radiation to penetrate the skin. A product that contains zinc oxide does provide blocking (reflective) capabilities but even zinc oxide, unless applied as a paste, allows a little UV light to penetrate the skin. For this reason, dermatologists recommended coupling sunscreen use with the wearing of sun protective clothing rated at UPF 50+ (which is the equivalent to a SPF 30 sunscreen).

Making a real fashion statement with sun protective clothing

With all of us feverishly trying to keep up with the latest fads Hollywood exports, finally there is a fashion tip that will truly enhance our lives.

Tom Cruise's former sidekick, Australian-raised actress Nicole Kidman, has often been quoted by the Associated Press as saying: "I wish that I hadn't been born with red hair and fair skin" as she is concerned about sun exposure and its direct link to an increased risk for skin cancer. She should know, too. After all, she hails from Australia where skin cancer is an exploding epidemic. Subsequently, Australia is the leading the world in heightening the quality of skin cancer prevention education and proactive sun safety behavior. Truth be told, skin cancer is the world's most common cancer. And Americans are no exception to the rule. Every hour someone in the United States dies from skin cancer, according to the American Academy of Dermatology. Perhaps, Kidman's example will encourage the propagation of a new fashion wave—sun protective clothing.

Whereas, sun protective clothing (also known as ultraviolet radiation protective clothing; or "UVR") is widely used in Australia, Europe, and South Africa, it is still relatively unknown here in the U.S. Sun protective clothing, however, is a highly effective option for individuals to protect themselves from the harmful affects of ultraviolet radiation all day, every day. If you consider that the average white 100% cotton T-shirt is equivalent to only a SPF 6 (which provides about 14% worth of sun protection), clearly there is a need for a light-weight, functional, stylish, economical, clothing that also provides exceptional protection from the sun.

Consequently, sun protective clothing blocks out more than 97.5% of UV rays (which is an equivalent to a SPF 30 sunscreen). This is considered by the Skin Cancer Foundation to be "the best of the best" when it comes to effective sun protection. If you consider that a SPF 20 sunscreen is 95% protective, than sun protective clothing is quite simply the most revolutionary new product available on the market today for those looking for a viable, yet extremely effective, way to protect themselves and their loved ones from sun damage. Dermatologist-oncologist, Sancy A. Leachman of the Tom C. Mathews Jr. Familial Melanoma Research Clinic at Huntsman Cancer Institute recommends that everyone use a sunscreen with a sun protection factor of 15 for daily, year-round use; SPF 30 is recommended if we are outdoors between 10:00 a.m. -and- 4:00 p.m. when UV rays are most intense. SPF 30 sunscreen is also highly recommended for those of us who possess multiple risk factors for skin cancer such as blonde or red hair, blue or green eyes, fair or sensitive skin, numerous atypical moles, and family history of skin cancer. Wearing sun protective clothing, coupled with proper year-round use of sunscreens, is the quite simply the best protection available, according to Leachman. And her colleagues in the field of dermatologic care agree.

"Appropriate sun apparel should offer effective protection against both short term and long term photo damage [such as wrinkling, skin cancer, and even cataracts]," says Dr. J.M. Mentor, a professor of dermatology at the Morehouse School of Medicine. In other words, effective sun safety apparel ought to protect against both UV-B and UV-A rays, and sun protective products such as those specially manufactured by Stingray® in Australia, (and distributed by various U.S. outlets such as SunSavvy.net) do exactly that.

Stingray® is the original sun protection clothing company to specialize in UV protection swimwear and daily attire for children and adults. "As a result of listening to the needs of our many customers, we are able to deliver products that take the 'sting out of the sun's rays,'" says Wendy Lister, Managing Director of Stingray®. "[People] are now getting the best possible UV protection." And now Americans also have access to this essential UV protection.

Glen and Liisa Thomson, both natives of South Africa, who now reside in Utah, a know first-hand the devastating toll sun damage can take on our health.

"We see a great and pressing need for increased awareness and education here in the U.S.," says Glen. "Too many times my wife and I will be at the pool, and see all these children running around sun burnt. Often, we'll offer shade and sunscreen to the parents so they can better protect their children." Glen and Liisa, are parents of two young children and realize the importance of instilling the practice of sunscreen usage and the wearing of sun protective clothing at a young age so as to develop a lifelong habit of sun safety behavior. In fact, the American Academy of Dermatology reports that sustaining just one severe "blistering" sunburn before age 18 increases one's likeliness of a future skin cancer diagnosis by an estimated 60%. This is of particular concern in states such as Colorado and Utah where high elevation exposes residents to more intense UV irradiation. Dr. Leachman explains it best by saying, "Someone standing on the summit of Mt. Timpanogos [Utah] will burn 66-to-77 times faster than someone standing on a beach in Los Angeles [California]." Lechman adds, "Skin cancer incidence is increasing at an alarming rate here in the United States, so it is important that we all take proper precautions to protect ourselves." The AAD solidifies Leachman's remarks, reporting 1.3-million Americans will be diagnosed with some form of skin cancer this year. "The risk is real," Leachman says. "There is a real need for people to take necessary precautions and to teach patients how to advocate for themselves [in reducing their risk for skin cancer]."

Accordingly, to further emphasize the importance of proper sun protection; properly applying sunscreen each day coupled with the wearing of UVR clothing, let us examine how ultraviolet radiation works, in doing so gain a deeper understanding of the relationship between exposure to ultraviolet radiation and the risk for developing skin cancer.

Understanding Ultraviolet Radiation:

- **What is solar ultraviolet radiation?** Ultraviolet radiation is defined as the portion of the electromagnetic spectrum between 100 nanometers (nm) and 400nm. Ultraviolet radiation is classified by wavelength into three regions: UV-A-Ultraviolet radiation in the range 315nm to 400nm is thought to contribute to premature aging and wrinkling of the skin and has recently been implicated as a cause of skin cancer. UV-B-ultraviolet radiation in the range 280nm to 315nm is more dangerous than UV-A, and has been implicated as the major cause of skin cancers, sun burns, and cataracts. UV-C-ultraviolet radiation in the range 100nm to 280nm is extremely dangerous but does not reach the earth's surface due to absorption in the atmosphere by the ozone layer.

- **How is ultraviolet radiation measured?** Broadband UV biometers and pyranometers are generally used to measure or monitor ultraviolet radiation. These instruments measure global ultraviolet radiation received on a horizontal surface from the entire hemisphere of the sky. Solar radiation includes both ultraviolet transmitted directly and scattered ultraviolet from the atmosphere so the design of these instruments ensures measurement of both direct and diffuse radiation. These instruments can also be used to monitor changes in ozone levels and cloud cover effects by measuring changes in ultraviolet irradiance levels.

- **What are the effects of exposure to ultraviolet radiation?** The major organs at risk from exposure to ultraviolet radiation are the skin and eyes as the penetration depth of ultraviolet radiation is very short. Ultraviolet radiation can be produced by various artificial sources but for most people the sun is the predominant source of ultraviolet radiation exposure. For outdoor workers without adequate protection or control measures the levels of solar ultraviolet radiation may exceed the generally accepted exposure limits. Those who have been over-exposed to ultraviolet radiation may be unaware of their injury as ultraviolet radiation cannot be seen or felt and does not produce an immediate reaction. Over-exposure to ultraviolet radiation can cause sunburn, skin damage and skin cancer. The most obvious short-term effect of over-exposure to ultraviolet radiation is sunburn. The more ultraviolet exposure, the worse the sunburn becomes. A person's cumulative exposure to ultraviolet along with the number of severe sunburns they have received, especially during childhood, increases their risk of developing skin cancer. Sun exposure causes the outer layers of the skin to thicken and long-term exposure can cause skin to wrinkle, sag and become leathery. Melanoma, the least common of the skin cancers but the most dangerous, may be related to severe exposure to ultraviolet radiation at an early age. Malignant melanomas may appear without warning as a dark mole or a dark "spot" on the skin. Ultraviolet radiation exposure also places our eyes at risk of photokeratitis, photoconjunctivitus and cataracts. Cataracts is the clouding of the lens of the eye, which is responsible for focusing light and producing sharp images. Without intervention cataracts can lead to blindness. There is also the risk for ocular melanoma, which is skin cancer on/or or near the eye.

- **How can I reduce my risk from exposure to ultraviolet radiation?** Increasing public awareness and interest in UV protection; educating people about proper methods of protecting themselves from skin cancer is imperative. Many forms of personal protection are available to reduce one's exposure to ultraviolet radiation. The best protection is to seek shade during the peak hours of 10:00 a.m. -and- 4:00 p.m. when ultraviolet radiation from the sun is strongest. When outdoors, wear sun protecting clothing with good body coverage (that is rated at UPF 50+), a wide-brimmed hat, UV protective wrap-around sunglasses and a SPF 15 sunscreen..

- **What is the UV Index?** Over-exposure to ultraviolet radiation can cause immediate effects such as sunburn coupled with long-term problems such as skin cancer and cataracts. The UV Index, which was developed by the National Weather Service and the U.S. Environmental Protection Agency (EPA), provides important information to help you plan your outdoor activities so as to prevent over-exposure to UV rays. The UV Index provides a daily forecast of the expected risk of overexposure to the sun. The Index predicts UV intensity levels on a scale of 1 to 11+, where low indicates a minimal risk of overexposure and 11+ means an extreme risk. Calculated on a next-day basis for every ZIP code across the United States, the UV Index takes into account clouds and other local conditions that affect the amount of UV radiation reaching the ground in different parts of the country.

UV Index Number	Exposure Level
0 to 2	Low
3 to 5	Moderate
6 to 8	High
8 to 10	Very High
11+	Extreme

Moreover, the American Academy of Dermatology asserts that nearly 90% of skin carcinomas are a result of over-exposure to UV rays. This, then, leads us to examine, more closely, the issue of tanning beds. The issue with regard to the use of artificial tanning lamps and tanning beds, and how increased popularity of such have contributed to the rising melanoma incidence, predominately among women in their 20s, is hotly debated. Controversy perpetuated by the media in recent years has since prompted the World Health Organization and the AAD to furnish public statements about the evidentiary dangers of using tanning beds. Since ultraviolet radiation is listed as a known carcinogen by the Centers for Disease Control and Prevention and Food and Drug Administration, and tanning beds emit ultraviolet radiation it is reasonable to conclude that tanning beds increase one's risk for skin cancer, particularly melanoma, which is the deadliest form. As a matter of fact, a recent study, issued in November 2006, was conducted by the International Agency for Research on Cancer Working Group regarding artificial ultraviolet (UV) light and skin cancer and solidifies the aforementioned. The abstract of that study reads as follows:

"Exposure to solar ultraviolet (UV) radiation is a known cause of skin cancer. Sunbed use represents an increasingly frequent source of artificial UV exposure in light-skinned populations. To assess the available evidence of the association between sunbed use and cutaneous malignant melanoma (melanoma) and other skin cancers, a systematic review of the literature until March 2006 on epidemiological and biological studies on sunbed use was performed in Pubmed, ISI Web of Science, Embase, Pascal, Cochrane library, Lilacs and Medcarib. Search for keywords in the title and in the abstract was done systematically and supplemented by manual searches. Only case-control, cohort or cross-sectional studies were selected. Data were abstracted by means of a standardized data-collection protocol. Based on 19 informative studies, ever-use of sunbeds was positively associated with melanoma (summary relative risk, 1.15; 95% CI, 1.00-1.31), although there was no consistent evidence of a dose-response relationship. First exposure to sunbeds before 35 years of age significantly increased the risk of melanoma, based on seven informative studies (summary relative risk, 1.75; 95% CI, 1.35-2.26). The summary relative risk of three studies of squamous cell carcinoma showed an increased risk. For basal cell carcinoma, the studies did not support an association. The evidence does not support a protective effect of the use of sunbeds against damage to the skin from subsequent sun exposure. Young adults should be discouraged from using indoor tanning equipment and restricted access to sunbeds by minors should be strongly considered" (Wiley-Liss).

Notably, the study indicates that "ever-use of sunbeds was positively associated with melanoma" and that "First exposure to sunbeds before 35 years of age significantly increased the risk of melanoma." Furthermore, the study suggests that "Young adults should be discouraged from using indoor tanning equipment and restricted access to sunbeds by minors should be strongly considered". I, as a skin cancer educator, would take that a step further and say that measures ought to be implemented to prohibit minors, under the age of 18, from using tanning beds.

In January 2007, Valerie Guild of the Charlie Guild Melanoma Foundation in California, and I fought for a bill in Utah, (where I run The Cancer Crusaders Organization), that asked for such a regulation. The bill, known as SB 52, called for minors to obtain parental consent. SB 52 was the first step toward protecting our young adults from the devastation of melanoma. Valerie's daughter, Charlie, was 25-years-old when she succumbed to melanoma. As such, I realize there remains much work yet to be done. Another colleague, Colette Coyne, who lost her 29-year-old daughter to melanoma, has fought for, and secured, legislation in New York to protect minors from tanning beds. In the meantime, rooting out the problem is a key to obtaining further understanding. We need to better understand why young adults desire to frequent tanning beds.

We, at The Cancer Crusaders Organization, conducted two random polls of 1,000 college-aged students (17-to-30) from March 2005 until August 2006, and discovered that an average 92% reported having used a tanning bed at least once in their lifetime. After having been apprised of the risks and dangers associated with tanning, many young adults remained undeterred. One of the first people we interviewed was my friend Erika Stevens, a graduate of Weber State University. "Not only does tanning help with my acne, it helps me feel good—makes me look and feel healthy," she said. "Even though, I am aware of the dangers of tanning, there is still that temptation; I haven't stopped using tanning beds and I never use sunscreens." More than a year since that first interview, Erika, in a recent follow-up, declared that she has since ceased to use tanning beds. "I use tanning foams now, Danielle! And that is the truth! I promise!"

Fortunately, continuous educational messages helped Erika; however, there are numerous young adults who have yet to forego their tanning habit. In point of fact are the words of Jen Slusser, a student at Brigham Young University who told the campus newspaper, *The Daily Universe* last year that she is aware of the risks but continues to frequent tanning beds. "I always feel it looks better being tan," she said. "Nowadays, a tan is equivalent to good looks." Such statements are akin to those generated by the American Academy of Dermatology.

The American Academy of Dermatology, in a 2006 survey, found that 80% of adolescents between the ages of 12-and-17 report being keenly aware of the risks of sun exposure and how such often leads to skin cancer; however, more than 66% of the teenagers that were interviewed said they look better with a tan and nearly half the teens said tans made them look healthier. "I hate looking deathly pale," 17-year-old Lindsay Vitez told the AAD. Vitez seeks a tan year-round, baking herself golden-brown at the tanning salons during the winter months and hanging out by the pool or in the summertime. Furthermore, she uses lotion to attract the sun, not protect against skin cancer, which is the least of her concerns. "I think a lot of teenagers realize it's dangerous, but because we're so wrapped up in the instant gratification we don't really worry about it," she said. And those feelings of instant gratification are coming at a particularly high price.

While the media continually propagates the "bronze look" as the "in look," an individual buying into this often pays with their life. In truth, the numbers of skin cancer incidents that occur each year far surpass that of all other cancers combined. More than 1.3 million Americans will be diagnosed with a form of skin cancer this year, according to the AAD. While in decades previous, melanomas did not typically occur in young adults in their 20s, that has dramatically changed and continues to rapidly. As mentioned previously, melanoma is now the most common form of cancer among women in their 20s. The American Cancer Society reports that people aged 35 or younger, who use tanning beds intermittently more than triple their chances of developing melanoma as compared to those who have never used tanning beds. This fact was re-emphasized and reiterated by the International Agency for Research on Cancer Working Group study referenced earlier.

"As college students and young adults, we sometimes think that we're invincible, or that cancer is an older person's disease," says Natalie Johnson, creator of the national Skin Cancer Awareness symbol and co-founder of The Cancer Crusaders Organization. Johnson is also a trained mole-mapping technician and has worked in the high-risk melanoma unit at Huntsman Cancer Institute. Natalie, a former Miss Utah, who lost her 21-year-old brother, Eric, to complications associated with a malignant melanoma, has taught more than 500,000 Utahns about the dangers of tanning. "I want to tell people that this [melanoma] is something that can affect anyone, no matter the age," she said.

In essence, avoid the use of tanning beds. *There is no such thing as a safe tan from a tanning bed.* Tanning is not a viable method of treating acne or seasonal depression, or any other health-related condition. And none of the countless e-mails I, or any of the other skin cancer advocates I work with, receive from the tanning industry requesting that we refrain from detailing the risks and dangers of tanning, will change this fact. It is not our intention to attack the indoor tanning industry nor any specific individual within that industry; rather our objective is to educate and protect our youth from a melanoma diagnosis. It is scientifically impossible to receive a tan from a tanning bed, or other forms of ultraviolet radiation, without sustaining measurable damage to your skin. Ultraviolet radiation is a known carcinogen that disrupts normal cell function, leading to damaged DNA, which can (and does) lead to cancer. Illustrating this fact is the following graphic courtesy of the *Deseret Morning News.*

Tanning beds
HOW THEY WORK

Tanning beds use long tubes containing inert gases, phosphorous coating and traces of mercury.

Electricity causes mercury atoms to lose their stability and emit energy in the form of UV radiation that stimulates the tanning process.

Tanning occurs on the epidermis

■ UVB light stimulates melanocytes to produce a pigment called melanin.

■ Melanin is oxidized by UVA light, darkening the skin.

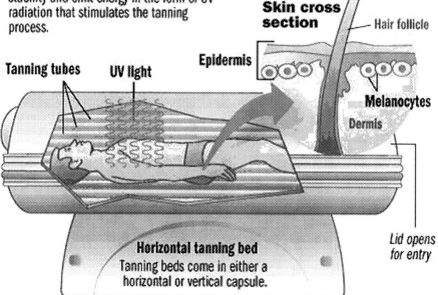

Skin cross section — Hair follicle

Epidermis

Melanocytes

Dermis

Tanning tubes **UV light**

Horizontal tanning bed
Tanning beds come in either a horizontal or vertical capsule.

Lid opens for entry

NOTE: vertical version tends to be stronger and produces a more even tan.

Although everyone has the same number of melanocytes (5 million), genetics determine how quickly an individual will tan.

SOURCE: tanning.gb.net

Therefore, if you could remove a cancer risk factor from your life, why not do it? Our genetic pre-disposition for numerous abnormal moles, our red/blonde hair and light eyes, are factors beyond our realm of control; however limiting our exposure to ultra-violet radiation is within our realm of control. We, as individuals, are our own best advocates in protecting ourselves and our loved ones from the devastating, adverse affects of skin cancer. The question now is: Are we willing to squelch our seemingly innate human desire to be popular? Are we to become slaves to vanity? After all, skin cancer is the most preventable of all cancer, despite it also being the world's most common cancer. We have the power to combat and eradicate this disease. And so the fight rages on, until victory is ours.

PART III

A) Programs in High-Risk States

- Arizona
- California
- Colorado
- Florida
- Texas
- Utah

B) National Organizations

- American Academy of Dermatology
- National Council on Skin Cancer Prevention
- Skin Cancer Foundation
- Sun Safety Alliance
- United States Environmental Protection Agency

ARIZONA

Arizona is known for its almost ever-present hot, sizzling sun. Two of my fellow board members at The Cancer Crusaders Organization can attest to this quite well. Margaret, who serves as our education consultant, served an 18-month mission for her church in Arizona where she hiked up and down the streets of Phoenix for 12-hours-a-day feeling as though she was "going to melt away in the Arizona sun." And, John, vice president, recently moved to Mesa with his wife and baby has shared similar such sentiments. Even Shonda Shilling, founder of the SHADE Foundation of America in Scottsdale, admits that when her baseball star husband, Curt, was transferred to Arizona (from Maryland) to play for the Arizona Diamondbacks, she was eager to soak up "almost completely unfiltered rays from the sun"; however, shortly after moving her young and growing family to Arizona, Shonda was diagnosed with a Stage II malignant melanoma. Shonda was 33-years-old. Shonda's lifelong love for sun tanning nearly cost Shonda her life.

Alas, Shonda's case is not a fluke or a phenomenon. Take, for instance, the story of 19-year-old Jacky Sims. Jacky, at age 15, had a malignant melanoma removed from her chest. Now in remission, Jacky volunteers with the SHADE Foundation teaching teenagers about the importance of sunscreen and sun protection, especially since less than 35% of young adults in Arizona (under the age of 25) use sunscreen, according to the American Cancer Society. And sun protection is of particular importance for Arizona residents.

The National Cancer Institute reports that Arizona has the second highest skin cancer incidence in the world after Australia. With more than 300 days of sunshine (compared to the national average of 200), Arizona residents are continually at higher-risk for skin cancer, even melanoma—the deadliest form. There were 851 people in Arizona diagnosed with melanoma last year. This year, in 2007, the Centers for Disease Control and Prevention (CDC) expect that over 940 people will be diagnosed. It is estimated that 23,560 new cases of non-melanoma skin cancer (basal-cell and squamous-cell carcinoma) will develop in 2007. Of those diagnosed, 9,710 will result in death.

This particularly high risk has resulted in the development of several programs to teach Arizonians about the importance of proper sun safety, particularly elementary school children whose sensitive skin pose an increased susceptibility to sunburn and sun damage.

As such, we have compiled a list of credible programs, approved by the American Academy of Dermatology, that are currently available—everything from how to obtain a grant to build a shade structure on your community soccer field, to fun and clever ways to teach your children about the UV index is included. For more information about your risk for melanoma and to schedule an appointment for your yearly skin cancer screening, we recommend contacting the Arizona Cancer Center which is National Cancer Institute-accredited facility.

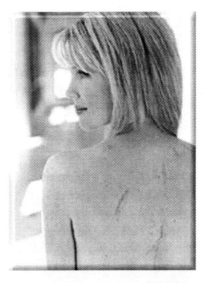

Shonda shortly after having five melanoma in-situs removed
from her back, chest, arms and legs.
Photo courtesy of Glamour Magazine and the SHADE Foundation.
© Glamour Magazine.

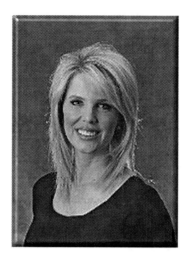

Today Shonda, a wife and mother of four, is cancer-free.
Photo taken by Rich Pilling.
© MLB. Photo courtesy of the SHADE Foundation.

Arizona Melanoma Organizations

SHADE Foundation of America

Mission Statement/Objectives:
To eradicate melanoma through the education of children and the community in the prevention and detection of skin cancer and the promotion of sun safety. To protect, educate,
encourage, and implement appropriate sun safety policies to assist schools in developing
and implementing a program to ensure all children spend their days in a SunWise® environment.

Founders (or Directors):
Curt Schilling, Shonda Schilling, and Sue Gorham

Point of Contact:
Sue Gorham, Executive Director

Full Mailing Address:
10510 N. 92nd Street
Scottsdale, Arizona 85258

Phone:
(480) 614-2278

E-mail Address and Web-site:
Sue@Shadefoundation.org; www.shadefoundation.org

Are you a 501 [c] [3] & is your status current? Yes

Date Founded: 2002

On-going Programs:
SHADE Foundation of America's SHADE grant program has approved grants for 81 shade
structures.

SHADE Foundation of America

<u>Additional Services Provided:</u>
Prevention and early detection are key issues in dealing with skin cancer. Most skin cancers are preventable, and if found early, treatable. The importance of screenings is growing as skin cancer is the fastest growing cancer of all cancers. During the past 4 years, over 5,000 people have been screened in SHADE sponsored and co-sponsored screenings. Free screenings are conducted by dermatologists and their staff. SHADE Foundation free screenings have taken place in many parts of the United States including Arizona, California, Florida, Massachusetts, and Tennessee.

<u>Affiliations:</u>
National Coalition for Sun Safety; National Council on Skin Cancer Prevention; EPA Sun-Wise; the Centers for Disease Control and Prevention (CDC).

The Phillips R. Geraghty Memorial Charity

<u>Mission/Objectives:</u>
The Phillips R. Geraghty Memorial Charity aims to increase awareness about the dangers of sun exposure and to encourage healthy sun habits among golfers. Through the tournament and a silent auction, the event will also raise money for the SHADE Foundation of America, a Phoenix-based organization dedicated to the eradication of skin cancer through education.

<u>Founders (or Directors):</u>
Laurel Naverson Geraghty and James P. Geraghty

<u>Date Founded:</u> March 18, 2006

<u>Point of Contact:</u>
Laurel Naversen Geraghty

<u>Full Mailing Address:</u>
5901 W. Behrend Drive Apt. 3010
Glendale, Arizona 85308

<u>E-mail Address and Web-site:</u>
lsnav@aol.com; www.shadefoundation.org/geraghty_golf.php

<u>Are you a 501 [c] [3] non-profit in good standing?</u> We are a fundraiser for the SHADE Foundation of America, a solidified 501 [c] [3]

<u>Sources of funding:</u>
100% Fundraising

<u>Affiliations:</u>
National Coalition for Sun Safety.

Arizona Cancer Centers

Arizona Cancer Center
c/o University of Arizona
Atten: David S. Alberts, M.D.
1501 North Campbell Avenue
Tucson, Arizona 85724
Phone: (520) 626-7925
Fax: (520) 626-2284

CALIFORNIA

As I write the introduction for my native state, I cannot help but sing that familiar classic made popular by The Mamas & The Papas entitled *"California Dreamin'."* It was recorded before I was born, but it is impossible to be raised in California and not hear that song or even be coerced into playing it for a middle school band recital. And, while it has been nearly a decade since I lived in California (I was raised in San Diego), my heart still holds a very special place for the Golden State. It is where I, as a 15-year-old orphan, stood on a bitter cold January day at the base of a fledgling evergreen, and felt my mother's velvety grey ashes slip through my fingers.

Speaking of the Golden State—When talking about skin cancer that phrase takes on an entirely different meaning for me. As many of you may already know, California got its nickname during the Gold Rush of the mid 1800s; however, after researching California's melanoma incidence and mortality rate, it would appear that its Hollywood golden girls (and boys) are paying the price for their love affair with the sun. And, I must admit that I was once a member of that club. While growing up, I lived to be outside in the warm year-round 80-degree weather. Though, my classmates in elementary school would jokingly chime the rhyme "Danielle White is so white she needs a tan," I was a very tan little girl with white blonde hair, blue eyes, and freckles dotting her nose. Truth be told, I was known to drench my Irish skin in baby oil so as to achieve a crisper, richer shade of tan. Examining pictures taken from my childhood, it is evident that I loved to play volleyball and go swimming, as many other Californians do. Yet, this over-exposure to ultraviolet radiation from the sun is catching up with us California die-hards.

Bringing this point into a sharper perspective, I am reminded of Charlie Guild. Charlie, a vibrant, talented, and lively young woman; the daughter of my friend and colleague Valerie Guild, was 25-years-old when melanoma robbed her of a rich life filled with limitless possibilities. It is distresses me that, at age 27, I have outlived not only Charlie, but several other peers who valiantly battled this insidious disease. Melanoma is an unnecessary epidemic; however, it continues to steal from us our friends and peers; our would-be parents, leaders, and teachers—our future.

Recently, I received an email from a colleague at the Environmental Protection Agency that stated of the six cancers of most concern "skin cancer incidence [and mortality] continues to rise." In fact, American Cancer Society estimates that more than 7,000 Californians will be diagnosed with melanoma in 2007. Comparatively, the American Academy of Dermatology reports that nearly 8,000 Americans will succumb to melanoma this year. Clearly, there is a pressing need for sun safe programs and policies in California. Fortunately, we, at The Cancer Crusaders Organization, work with many of those who are spearheading these programs and have listed them here in this section.

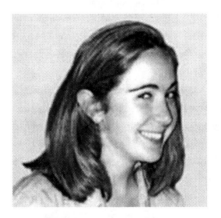

Charlie Guild was diagnosed with malignant melanoma at age 25 and passed away just eight months after her initial diagnosis.
Photo courtesy of the Charlie Guild Melanoma Foundation.

California Melanoma Organizations

American Melanoma Foundation

Mission Statement/Objectives:
The American Melanoma Foundation is a voluntary health agency, registered as a 501[c] [3] charitable, non-profit organization. AMF is governed by a volunteer Board of Directors dedicated to serving the needs of patients and communities nationwide, and is a member of the National Council on Skin Cancer Prevention.

Founders (or Directors):
Dr. Mona Mofid

Point of Contact:
Dr. Mona Mofid, Director

Full Mailing Address:
12395 El Camino Real, Suite 117
San Diego, California 92130

Phone:
(619) 448-0991

E-mail Address and Web-site:
admin@sandiegoskin.com; www.melanomafoundation.org

Are you a 501 [c] [3] non-profit organization & is your status current? Yes

Date Founded: 1990

Sources of funding:
100% Donations & Fundraising

Annual Events:
AMF Sun Awareness Day; SunWise Poster Contest; SunSmart Games Day.

On-going Programs:
Monthly Melanoma Patient Support Group.

Additional Services Provided:
Clinical oncology trials in cooperation with the National Institutes of Health; patient bookstore.

American Melanoma Foundation

Affiliations:
National Council on Skin Cancer Prevention; "ONE VOICE" for Melanoma.

Charlie Guild Melanoma Foundation

Mission Statement/Objectives:
Our mission at the Charlie Guild Melanoma Foundation is to raise awareness and prevent melanoma through legislative efforts and physician education, increase research efforts and aid in the rapid approval of new drugs.

Founders (or Directors):
Valerie Guild

Point of Contact:
Valerie Guild, Executive Director

Full Mailing Address:
85 Seafirth Road
Tiburon, California 94920

Phone and Fax:
Phone: (415) 305-0060; Fax (510) 235-8002

E-mail Address and Web-site:
vguild@charlie.org; www.charlie.org

Are you a 501 [c] [3] & is your status current? Yes

Date Founded: 2004

Sources of funding: 90% Grants; 10% Donations

Annual Events:
International Melanoma Working Group.

On-going Programs:
K-12 Mandatory Sun Safety Education Legislation, and Indoor Tanning Legislation.

Additional Services Provided:
Consult with legislators throughout the United States regarding sun safety education.

Affiliations:
National Council on Skin Cancer Prevention; "ONE VOICE" for Melanoma.

Noteworthy Awards/Recognitions:
Our founder, Valerie Guild, was named 2006 "Cancer Crusader of the Year" by The Cancer Crusaders Organization and SunSavvy, LLC.

Charlie Guild Melanoma Foundation

Misc:
Led indoor tanning legislation under consideration in New York, Connecticut, Washington, California, Maryland, Massachusetts, and Minnesota;
Led legislation mandating K-12 sun safety education, and/or similar education for outdoor workers passed or pending in New York, Texas, California, Florida, Washington, Utah, Connecticut, Kentucky, Pennsylvania, Maryland and Massachusetts;
Initiated the established of a melanoma tissue bank with the participation of the United States Military, University of California San Francisco, Huntsman Cancer Institute in Salt Lake City, Utah, and the University of Pittsburgh Cancer Institute;
Creation of the International Melanoma Working Group, the first international melanoma conference, to held in Germany in 2006;
Initiated the creation of a computer-based training seminar geared to pediatricians/pediatric residents in the area of childhood skin cancer prevention.

Melanoma Research Foundation

Mission/Objectives:
To support medical research for finding effective treatments and eventually a cure for melanoma; To educate patients and physicians about the prevention, diagnosis and treatment of melanoma; To act as an advocate for the melanoma community to raise the awareness of this disease and the need for a cure.

Founders (or Directors):
Diana Ashby and Linda Pilkington

Point of Contact:
Randy Lomax, California branch

Date Founded: 1996

Full Mailing Address:
493 La Prenda Road
Los Altos, California 94024

Phone:
1.800.MRF.1290

E-mail Address and Web-site:
lomax@jps.net; **www.melanoma.org**

Are you a 501 [c] [3] non-profit in good standing? Yes

Sources of funding:
33% Donations/Membership Dues; 56% Fundraising; 11% Grants & Corporate Sponsorships

Melanoma Research Foundation

Annual Events:
Celebrity Golf Tournament in Tarzana, California.

Additional Services Provided:
Patient and Caregiver support and education via the Melanoma Patient Information Page (www.mpip.org) and our toll-free support hotline; Assistance with grass roots events and activities such as "ONE VOICE" Melanoma Network.

Noteworthy Awards & Recognitions:
The MRF was instrumental in organizing the first "ONE VOICE" Melanoma Network meeting in March 2006 at the National Institutes of Health, which brought together all melanoma-specific foundations. The MRF also was instrumental in forming the Society of Melanoma Researchers, which is now a very active organization of melanoma researchers.

Affiliations:
National Council on Skin Cancer Prevention.

National Melanoma Awareness Project

Mission Statement/Objectives:
Our goals are: To provide a network for collaboration on national skin cancer educational outreach efforts; To educate the community about the realities of skin cancer, with emphasis on prevention and early detection of melanoma through sun protection and frequent self-screening; To leave students with an interest in teaching their friends and loved ones about melanoma; To increase awareness, knowledge, and suspicion of melanoma in future physicians across all medical specialties; To personalize teaching about melanoma and to connect those affected by it through sharing of real-life stories.

Founders (or Directors):
Jeanette Waller

Point of Contact:
Jeanette Waller and William Rietkerk

Full Mailing Address:
National Melanoma Awareness Project
University of California, Irvine Dept of Dermatology
C340, Medical Sciences I
Irvine, California 92697-2400

Phone and Fax:
Phone: (949) 533-6892; Fax: (949) 856-1072

E-mail Address and Web-site:
info@spotaspot.org; jwaller@uci.edu; www.spotaspot.org

National Melanoma Awareness Project

Are you a 501 [c] [3] & is your status current? Pending

Date Founded: 2005

Sources of funding: 100% Donations

Annual Events:
Each medical school chapter at UC Irvine hosts an annual Volunteer Appreciation Luncheon every Spring.

On-going Programs:
We are continually working to recruit more medical schools to join in our efforts. At each medical school, student leaders are continually working to set up teaching sessions at local grade-schools. Generally, the teaching sessions are 45-50 minutes in duration, including interactive games that help solidify the students' knowledge and encourage them to share what they've learned. In order to make it easy for any medical school to participate, we provide the complete curriculum, with statistics and information customized to geographic area, in addition to standardized recruitment and informational letters to be used for establishing relationships with new grade-schools.

Additional Services Provided:
In addition to teaching the curriculum, we also host an annual poster contest; medical student volunteers bring flyers each time they teach in order to promote the poster contest. It is hoped that by creating posters to educate others about sun protection and skin cancer prevention and detection, students will feel some "ownership" of the message and of their role in sharing it. In many cases, with student and parent permission, posters may be replicated and posted around the local community to further increase awareness.

Affiliations:
National Council on Skin Prevention; "ONE VOICE" for Melanoma.

William S. Graham Foundation for Melanoma Research, Inc. (a.k.a. "Billy Foundation")

Mission Statement:
The primary activities of this 501 [c] [3] non-profit foundation are to educate the public regarding the cause and prevention of melanoma and through specific public awareness programs, assist in the early detection of this deadly cancer and to raise funds to assist the research for the cure.

Founders (or Directors):
Karen L. Graham

Point of Contact:
Susan Hollister, National Program Director

William S. Graham Foundation for Melanoma Research, Inc. (a.k.a. "Billy Foundation")

Full Mailing Address:
26203 Production Avenue #12A
Hayward, California 94545

Phone and Fax:
Phone: 1-888-88-BILLY, 510-264-9078; Fax: (510) 264-9079

E-mail Address and Web-site:

Are you a 501 [c] [3] non-profit and in good standing? Yes

Date Founded: 1996

Sources of Funding: 75% Corporate donations; 5% Individual donations; 20% Fundraising

Annual Events:
SunSafe Moonlit Night Gala Fundraising Event

On-going programs:
SS Kidz®—SS Kids sun safety education program developed for preschool through primary grades using interactive storylines, music and games for young children, and a slide presentation and open forum for grades 6-12. Using an interactive curriculum we draw the classroom/assembly into a colorful storyline of children, similar to themselves, and their adventures as they come in contact with familiar animals that teach them about Sun Safety Awareness. A diverse program is also available for middle school through high school using a slide show presentation and peer education.
Mole Patrol—Mole Patrol goes out into the community across the country offering free skin cancer screening and facts about sun safety. Board Certified Dermatologists volunteer their time for this program which has been sanctioned by the American Academy of Dermatology.
Legislation—Initiated and sponsored groundbreaking legislation in the U.S. "Billy's Bill for Sun Safety"; which granted children the use of hats and sunscreen on California school campuses (SB310 and SB1632).
Research—A Medical Advisory Committee assists in decisions regarding awarding research grants and scholarships, as well as assisting in keeping the foundation office up to date on the latest clinical trials, procedures and statistics. In coordination with the AACR, the "Billy Foundation" sponsored the first $30,000 Fellows Grant for Melanoma Research and in 2005 recently sponsored a first of its kind public forum at the 6th World Congress on Melanoma in 2005.

William S. Graham Foundation for Melanoma Research, Inc. (a.k.a. "Billy Foundation")

Additional Services Provided:
The foundation is also a strong and effective advocate for patients and families through an interactive Web-site, referrals, clinical trials matching service, and lobbying for patient rights and care. We use our 1-888-88-BILLY toll free number to assist patients and their families dealing with melanoma. Legislative involvement as leader authoring, and getting passed the first of its kind Sun Safety legislation in the USA. SB 310 and SB1632 now known as "Billy's Bill for Sun Safety."

Awards & Recognitions:
2001 American Academy of Dermatology Golden Triangle Award; 2002 Commendation from California Governor Gray Davis; Congressional Record in place at the National Library of Congress by Congressman, Pete Stark; Named 2006 "Organization of the Year" by The Cancer Crusaders Organization and SunSavvy, LLC.

Affiliations:
National Coalition for Sun Safety, National Council on Skin Cancer Prevention, "ONE VOICE" for Melanoma.

California Cancer Centers

Cancer Research Center
c/o The Burnham Institute
Atten: Kristiina Vuori, M.D., Ph.D.
10901 North Torrey Pines Road
La Jolla, California
Phone: (858) 646-3100; Fax: (858) 713-6272

Chao Family Comprehensive Cancer Center
c/o University of California at Irvine
Atten: Frank L. Meyskesn, Jr., M.D.
101 The City Drive
Bldg. 23, Route 81, Room 406
Orange, California 92868
Phone: (714) 456-6310; Fax: (714) 456-2240 (fax)

City of Hope National Medical Center
c/o Beckman Research Institute
1500 East Road

Duarte, California 91010
Phone: (626) 256-HOPE; Fax: (626) 930-5394

Jonsson Comprehensive Cancer Center
c/o University of California Los Angeles
Atten: Judith C. Gasson, Ph.D.
Facto Building #8-684
10833 Le Conte Avenue
Los Angeles, California 90095
Phone: (310) 825-5268; Fax (310) 206-5553

Norris Comprehensive Cancer Center
c/o University Southern California
Atten: Peter A. Jones, Ph.D.
1441 Eastlake Avenue, NOR 8392L
Los Angeles, California 90089
Phone: (323) 865-0816; Fax: (323) 865-0102

Rebecca and John Moores Cancer Center
c/o University of California at San Diego
Atten: Dennis A. Carson, M.D.
3855 Health Sciences Drive #2247
La Jolla, California 92093
Phone: (858) 822-1222; Fax: (858) 822-1207

Salk Institute Cancer Center
Atten: Walter Eckhard, Ph.D.
10010 North Torrey Pines Road
La Jolla, California 92037
Phone: (858) 453-4100 ext. 1386; Fax: (858) 457-4766

UC Davis Cancer Center
c/o University of California, Davis
Atten: Ralph W. deVere White, M.D.
4501 X Street #3003
Sacramento, California 95817
Phone: (916) 734-5800; Fax: (916) 451-4464

UCSF Comprehensive Cancer Center & Cancer Research Institute
c/o University of California San Francisco
Atten: Frank McCormick, Ph.D.
2350 Sutter Street, Box 0128
San Francisco, California 94115
Phone: (415) 502-1710; Fax: (415) 502-1712

COLORADO

"I remember sitting out there in the sun and putting baby oil on my skin," said LPGA star Jill McGill, to the press upon learning of her melanoma diagnosis. "It was that and growing up in that Colorado sun. Nobody thought about it in those days." Jill, who began golfing at age 12, was diagnosed with malignant melanoma at age 33. She discovered a "dark spot" on her left thigh in May 2004. When Jill realized that, after six months, the spot on her thigh was growing, she went into the dermatologist to have it examined. It was then that Jill was told that she needed to undergo surgery immediately. "I had a huge chunk cut out of my thigh," McGill says. Fortunately, Jill is alive and well, and still golfing. She now resides in San Diego with her husband.

Mark Goldman, also from Colorado, was told by doctors, in 1998, that he had a metastatic melanoma on his liver after "being assured that I would never be bothered by my early stage melanoma again." Mark was first diagnosed in 1990. Today, Mark is cancer-free after receiving treatment at the University of Colorado Health Sciences Center. He now works full-time for the National Coalition for Cancer Survivorships.

Bill Owens, former governor of Colorado, is, like Jill and Mark, now cancer-free and working to support skin cancer prevention education and melanoma research in his home state where the sun shines more than 300 days a year.

"Every year in Colorado, about 700 invasive melanomas are diagnosed and about 120 people will die of the disease. Given how treatable this cancer is in its early stages, this is tragic. With early detection and treatment, most forms of skin care are curable" said former Governor Bill Owens during the kick of "Skin Cancer Awareness" Month at the Colorado State Capitol in May 2006.

After Governor Owens gave the proclamation and shared his experience with battling skin cancer, I spoke with his dermatologist Dr. Gregory G. Papadeas, who practices at the Advanced Dermatology Skin and Laser Surgery Center in Aurora.

"In Colorado, the sun shines over 300 days a year," he said. Dr. Papadeas, who was raised in Denver, and has served as past president of the Colorado Dermatologic Society, knows how devastating a lifetime of unprotected sun can be on a person. "We [Colorado natives] are also at a very high altitude, which means that we are exposed to more ultraviolet rays. What's more, we are a very recreation-oriented state. All of these factors contribute to the high incidence of skin cancer in Colorado."

Colorado has a culmination of risk factors which include, as Dr. Papadeas mentioned, higher land elevation and above average number of days where the sun shines. Colorado, like Utah, also experiences a considerable amount of snowfall, and with approximately 30-to-60% of ultraviolet rays being reflective from snow, it places Colorado residents at an increased risk for skin cancer. Thusly, the concept of year-round sun protection is of paramount importance to Colorado residents. Enjoy the wide array of outdoor activities your state offers throughout the year, but consider the example of Mark, Jill, and Bill. Be SunSavvy®.

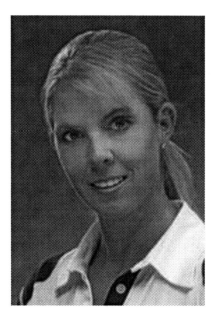

LPGA star, Jill McGill, from Colorado, was diagnosed with melanoma at age 33 when suspicious "dark spot" failed to heal after six months. Today Jill is cancer-free, and is careful to slather on sunscreen before hitting the green. *Photo courtesy of the LPGA. © LPGA.*

Colorado Melanoma Organizations

Colorado Skin Cancer Task Force

Mission Statement/Objectives:
The Colorado Skin Cancer Task, as part of the Colorado Cancer Coalition, coordinates statewide efforts to increase skin caner prevention practices and policies, and to reduce the morbidity and mortality of skin cancer in Colorado.

Points of Contact:
Colorado Cancer Coalition

Full Mailing Address:
4300 Cherry Creek Drive South A5
Denver, Colorado 80246

Phone and Fax:
Phone: (303) 692-2520; Fax: (303) 691-7721

Web-site:
www.coloradocancercoalition.org

Are you a 501 [c] [3] & is your status current? Yes. We are, in fact, a conglomerate of various health-related organizations throughout the State of Colorado.

On-going Programs:
Colorado State Cancer Control Plan for 2005-2010.

Additional Services Provided:
We are working on comprehensive, multi-channel state wise programs promotion skin cancer prevention through schools, pediatric and primary care clinics, and workplaces.

Affiliations:
Colorado Dermatologic Society; University of Colorado Cancer Center (Skin Cancer Research Clinic).

Colorado Cancer Centers

University of Colorado Cancer Center
Atten: Paul A. Bunn, Jr., M.D.

c/o University of Colorado Health Sciences Center
P.O. BOX 6511—Mail Stop #8111
Aurora, Colorado 80045
Phone: (303) 724-3155; Fax: (303) 315-2204

FLORIDA

When my friends and I were sending in our college application, I remember Janet and Levant praying to be accepted to a Florida school so that they would be in close proximity to a beach; "I could take my surf board with me to class," they said. I can still remember their shrieks and shrills of glee upon receiving their acceptance letters to the University of South Florida. At that time, we had never heard of this disease called "melanoma", and had little, if any, understanding of how over-exposure to ultraviolet radiation played a integral part in significantly increasing one's risk for skin cancer. As 17-year-olds attending an American high school in Japan, Janet and Levant decided that going to college in Florida meant they would have the best of both worlds—career advancement and limitless sunshine to satisfy their hunger for tropical paradise. Hence, the year-round sunshine is the reason why Florida has been given the nickname of "Sunshine State".

Being the Sunshine State, skin cancer in Florida is not merely a concern, but rather it is a harsh reality. It is a fact of life. According to the Florida Department Health, of the 1.3-million new skin cancers diagnosed in United States this year, more than 97,000 of those will be found among Florida residents. Of the 8,000 melanoma related deaths expected this year, 40,090 of those will occur in Florida.

"It is definitively a serious concern for us who live in Florida," wrote Governor Jeb Bush in an email to me last year. "The Florida Department of Health works hard to encourage everyone to not only protect their skin, but also to get screened for skin cancer."

In May 2006, I contacted all 50 U.S. Governors about skin cancer prevention programs/sun safety initiatives in their respective states. While on the phone with Governor Jeb Bush's office, discussing a proclamation declaring a state-wide celebration of national Skin Cancer Awareness month, the office manager shared her feelings about skin cancer, with great concern: "Skin cancer is a huge concern for all of us here in Florida [...] This is a pressing issue that requires the immediate attention of all concerned individuals in Florida, and throughout the United States. It is the fastest growing cancer [but] it is preventable," she said.

Several days after my conversation with Governor Bush's office, I received an email from my Grandma White who currently resides in Florida. (I have not seen her since 1995). Her email read as follows: "This is a most worthy endeavor. Grandpa and I make sure and visit the dermatologist quite regularly for skin screenings." I had to chuckle—*Well, it looks like the word got out in Florida!*

Certainly, fighting skin cancer is a worthwhile endeavor. In 2005, the <u>Journal of the American Academy of Dermatology</u> published an article that put it this way: "In light of the increasing frequency of skin cancer in younger adults, researchers emphasize the importance of skin-cancer prevention messages. Risk of skin cancer can be decreased by avoiding sun exposure, wearing sun-protective clothing and hats, and using sunscreen."

I hope that Janet and Levant, as they inhale the salty sea breeze on a beach somewhere in Florida, are armed with an ample supply of Blue Lizard Australian Suncream and therefore protecting themselves from the world's most common cancer.

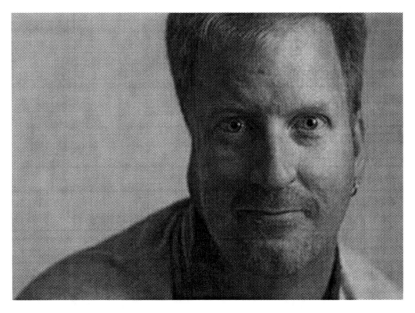

Scott Lindstam, at age 35, had his right ear amputated after it was discovered he his pesky sore was, in fact, invasive melanoma. *Photo courtesy of the St. Petersburg Times.* © *St. Petersburg Times.*

Apollo Sunguard Systems, Inc.

Mission/Objectives:
Apollo Sunguard Systems, Inc., manufactures shade structures that block more than 93% of UV radiation and has developed proprietary systems to shade playgrounds in Florida

Founders (or Directors):
Kevin Connelly

Point of Contact: Kevin Connelly, President

Full Mailing Address:
4487 Ashton Road
Sarasota, Florida 34233

Phone and Fax:
Phone: (941) 925-3000; Fax: (941) 925-3001

E-mail Address and Web-site:
president@sunguard.net; www.sunguard.net

Are you a 501 [c] [3] non-profit in good standing? Yes

Additional Services Provided:
Playground shades for parks and recreation facilities, schools, and daycare facilities.

Bill Walter III Melanoma Research Fund

Mission Statement/Objectives:
The vision and mission of the Bill Walter III Melanoma Research Fund is to help find a cure for melanoma by supporting promising melanoma research. The Fund also assists melanoma patients who are undergoing treatment, and endeavors to save lives by raising awareness of the dangers of melanoma.

Founders (or Directors):
The Bill Walter III Family and Friends

Point of Contact:
Dr. William A. Walter, Vice President

Bill Walter III Melanoma Research Fund

Phone and Fax:
Phone: (386) 257-5798; Fax: (386) 257-1585

E-mail Address and Web-site:
ALGrnd@aol.com; www.billwalteriii.org

Are you a 501 [c] [3] non-profit organization & is your status current? Yes

Date Founded: 1998

Sources of funding:
100% Donations & Fundraising

Annual Events:
Annual Bill Walter III Melanoma Research Fund 5K Run/Walk in Florida; Annual RayZ Awareness 5K Fundraiser in Colorado.

On-going Programs:
We, through donations, have provided more than $42,000 to financially assist melanoma patients around the country and have donated $100,000 for current melanoma research.

The Kristi Michael Memorial Foundation (a.k.a. "The Spirit of Kristi")

Mission Statement/Objectives:
The goals of The Spirit of Kristi are: To assist the families of patients undergoing clinical trials at the National Institutes of Health in Bethesda, Maryland.; To assist in the publics awareness of skin cancer prevention

Founders (or Directors):
Stan Kozmas

Point of Contact:
Stan Kozmas, Director

E-mail Address and Web-site:
info@thespiritofkristi.com; www.thespiritofkrisit.com; www.kristimichael.com

Are you a 501 [c] [3] non-profit organization & is your status current? Yes

Richard David Kann Melanoma Foundation

Mission Statement/Objectives:
The mission of the Richard David Kann Melanoma Foundation, a 501 [c] [3] not-for-profit organization, is to save lives by educating the public on sun safety and the prevention and early detection of skin cancer, especially melanoma

---

Richard David Kann Melanoma Foundation

Founders (or Directors):
Deborah Kann Schwarzberg and Dr. Jer Zeneiris

Point of Contact:
Tamika Peay, Executive Director

Full Mailing Address:
621 Clearwater Park Road
West Palm Beach, Florida 33401

Phone and Fax:
Phone: (561) 655-9655; Fax: (561) 655-9650

E-mail Address and Web-site:
info@melanomafoundation.org; www.melanomafoundation.org

Are you a 501 [c] [3] & is your status current? Yes

Date Founded: 1995

Sources of funding: 60% Grants; 20% Donations; 20% Fundraising

Annual Events:
Annual "SunSational" Luncheon & Fashion Show (February); Annual Golf Tournament (December); Annual Skin Cancer Awareness Day—"Melanoma Monday" (May).

On-going Programs:
The Foundation provides free presentations to schools, community organizations and corporations all over the country. This school-based teaching is provided with our K-12 curricula, SunSmart America™. SunSmart America™ meets existing requirements in science, math, health, and language arts for grades K-12. All take home activities are available in English, Spanish, Haitian Creole, and Portuguese. It has been implemented in schools all over the country and Canada.

Noteworthy Awards/Recognitions:
The Richard David Kann Melanoma Foundation, in collaboration with the University of Miami, received a grant from the National Cancer Institute of the National Institutes of Health for a 5-year longitudinal study to quantify the effectiveness of SunSmart America's™ Elementary School Curriculum. The Centers for Disease Control and Prevention featured SunSmart America™ with their on-line high school contest in 2002. The Foundation is a nine-time winner of the Gold Triangle Award from the American Academy of Dermatology (AAD).

Florida Cancer Centers

H. Lee Moffitt Cancer Center & Research Institute

c/o University of South Florida
Atten: William S. Dalton, M.D., Ph.D.
12902 Magnolia Drive, MCC-CEO
Tampa, Florida 33612
Phone: (813) 615-4261: Fax: (813) 615-4258 (fax)

TEXAS

A short time ago, I was flatly informed there is an un-written rule that states Texans and Californians cannot be friends, but as a California-raised woman, I must admit that I have never met a Texan that I did not like. Four of my college room-mates were from Texas, three other room-mates relocated to Texas after graduation, one room-mate recently married a Texan, my best friend hails from Texas, and one of my favorite dermatologists, Dr. Clay J. Cockerell, lives and practices in Texas. It is with good reason that Texans have pride for their "Lone Star State"—good people come from Texas. There are only two downsides to Texas. First, it is not California. Like California, however, Texas is considered a high risk state for skin cancer. In 1999, the year my co-founder lost her 21-year-old brother to melanoma, there were 2,900 melanoma incidents. The Texas Cancer Council expects that in 2007, there will be nearly 5,000 Texans diagnosed with melanoma.

As I write this, my thoughts and prayers are with the Zants family (the Zants are close family friends with my best friend, Melissa). I had the privilege of meeting the Zants' last summer while they were vacationing in Utah. They shared with me how melanoma has touched them. I can still remember the pain in their voice, the strength and passion behind their handshakes and hugs, and the pleading in their eyes. I think of the Zants' and pray for them often.

I also think about (and worry about) Melissa's dad, who spends his days running a successful pool cleaning business in the blazing Texas sun—

Is he slathering on the sunscreen? Is he using the right sunscreen- a broad-spectrum SPF 15+ formula? Should I send him more sunscreen? I'll have to send sunscreen home with Melissa next time she goes home to visit. Is he properly protected from sun? What about all that reflection that is coming off all of those pools? Please keep him safe from harm. Don't let skin cancer touch him, or his family. Please, Heavenly Father, I pray.

Conceivably the most famous Texan with skin cancer is First Lady Laura Bush who, in October 2006, told the Associated Press that she had squamous cell caricoma, a form of skin cancer, removed from her right leg. Bush thought the sore on her leg was an insect bite that had grown infected.

"Actually it never occurred to me to make it public," she said. "It was very minor. I thought it was an insect bite, actually, when I first got it, and then it just didn't get well." Bush added, "I was never sick. I never felt badly." She blamed the cancer on the hot west Texas sun and her fair complexion.

"I never did a lot of sun bathing like some my friends did, because I didn't tan, really," she said. "But of course I played outside for my whole childhood [and] spent afternoons at the swimming pool and did those things that we all did growing up in Texas, and so I was out in the sun a lot."

On the other hand, Karl Matthiessen was not as fortunate as the First Lady. Karl Matthiessen, the 2007 Dallas, Texas "Miles for Melanoma" Honoree, was a 38; a husband and father, when he lost his battle with the deadliest form of skin cancer. First diagnosed, on his 35th birthday, Karl's Stage III malignant melanoma quickly spread throughout his body and took him from his young family.

"He went through two brain surgeries, radiation and chemotherapy to kill the cancer," says his wife. "He was well respected and loved. At his work, the company flag flew at half mast for that week in October [2006] and more than 200 people attended his memorial. We hope that he's doing a lot of scuba diving, martini drinking and guitar playing in heaven. He is missed but always loved. He is the love of my life."

Once again, my thoughts and prayers are turned toward my best friend's father, the Zants', and all the families mentioned in this book.

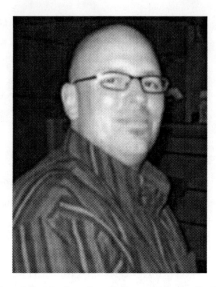

A loving husband and husband to Celine and Anika, Karl Matthiessen,
succumbed to melanoma on October 1, 2006. He was 38-years-old.
Photo courtesy of the James A. Schlipmann Melanoma Cancer Foundation.

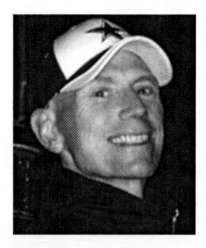

"First and foremost, Jim was a loving husband and daddy," says his wife
Shirley. James Janovsky battled melanoma for six continuous years. A
mole on his scalp was diagnosed as melanoma, and despite 13 surgeries,
James lost his valiant battle on September 14, 2006.
Photo courtesy of the James A. Schlipmann Melanoma Cancer Foundation.

James A. Schlipmann Melanoma Cancer Foundation (a.k.a. "The Schlip")

Mission Statement/Objectives:
Our mission at the James A. Schlipmann Melanoma Cancer Foundation is to fund clinical trials and research studies, to advance education, awareness, screenings, and treatment to eventually eradicate melanoma.

Founders (or Directors):
A. Jean Schlipmann

Point of Contact:
A. Jean Schlipmann, President

Full Mailing Address:
3217 Bob O Link Court
Plano, Texas 75093

Phone:
(972) 307-9325

E-mail Address and Web-site:
TheSchlip@tx.rr.com; www.TheSchlip.com

Are you a 501 [c] [3] non-profit organization & is your status current? Yes

Date Founded: 2002

Sources of funding: 15% Donations; 5% Grants; 80% Fundraising

Annual Events:
The Schlip Miles for Melanoma Walk in Texas, Florida, Illinois, Louisiana, Missouri, Maryland, and Ohio; The Schlip Golf Classic for Melanoma in Texas; The Schlip Poker Run for Melanoma in Illinois; The Schlip Bowl-A-Thon for Melanoma in New Hampshire and Illinois.

Additional Services Provided:
The Schlip Clinical Trial Matching Service.

Affiliations:
National Council on Skin Cancer Prevention; the World Community Grid—Cure Melanoma Team; "ONE VOICE" for Melanoma.

Texas Cancer Centers

M.D. Anderson Cancer Center
c/o University of Texas
Atten: John Mendelsohn, M.D.
1515 Holcombe Boulevard Box #91
Houston, Texas 77030
Phone: (713) 792-2121; Fax: (713) 799-2210

San Antonio Cancer Institute
c/o University of Texas Health Science Center at San Antonio
Atten: Thomas J. Slaga, Ph.D.
7703 Floyd Curl Drive, MSC 7772
San Antonio, Texas 78229
Phone: (210) 567-2710; Fax: (210) 567-2709

UTAH

With more than 224 days of sunshine, it's not California, but after eight years in Utah, it has become a part of me. Everyone I love currently lives in Utah. And, there is where I feel where I need to be at the present time, especially since Utah's risk for skin cancer is the highest in the nation—1 in 52 as compared to 1 in 65 nationally, according to Huntsman Cancer Institute.

In 2003, when my friend Natalie Camille Johnson was serving as Miss Utah, she presented the American Academy of Dermatology with the idea of a universally accepted and recognizable ribbon symbol representing Skin Cancer Awareness. Her original design featured an orange loop ribbon encompassing a yellow sunburst in the center. The AAD responded favorably to Natalie's proposal, and hence the National Skin Cancer Awareness Symbol© was born. At this time, there were 420 melanomas diagnosed in Utah. Four years later that number is expected to exceed 500.

Since teaming up with Natalie and establishing The Cancer Crusaders Organization, I have met literally, thousands of individuals, both in and outside of the State of Utah, who have been touched by skin cancer. Each person I come in contact with leaves an imprint upon my heart much akin to a fingerprint. It is as unique and easily identifiable, and ever-lasting. One of the many remarkable individuals who have impacted my life, and has since grown to become a dear friend, is Tiffany Berg.

Tiffany and I were introduced through a mutual friend during the summer of 2004. The Cancer Crusaders Organization was still a fledgling non-profit skin cancer education facility, but receiving a considerable amount of media attention with the launch of our *"Only Skin Deep?"*® campaign to introduce the new national Skin Cancer Awareness ribbon. Tiffany's husband, Paul, a father of five, was fighting squamous-cell carcinoma—for the second time—and since Tiffany was the host of a television program, she invited me to talk about sun safety with her viewers.

I can still remember our first telephone conversation. She and I talked as though we had been friends for years. We cried together. We prayed together. The sound of Tiffany's voice as she prayed for her husband, for their children, and for the success of Cancer Crusaders, remains with me. I can still remember the fluctuations of her voice, the pauses between words and phrases, and the feeling that filled the room. There we were, two women—practically strangers, praying to our Heavenly Father via the telephone wires. A few months after this took place, circumstances were as such that I found myself on the phone with Tiffany, once again, praying. She told me something that day, amid my unremitting tears, that has stayed with me. I find myself referring back to it, often.

"Danielle, if there is a lesson to be learned from cancer, it is that, while it is good and honorable to fight cancer, we must not forget to live. We can honor those who have gone before us; our loved ones that cancer has taken from us, but, we must not forget to live."

When Tiffany told me this, her husband's skin cancer, which began as a unrelenting sore on his lip, had returned and was now growing in the epithelial layer of his mouth, up through his nasal cavity, and heading toward his eyes. The Bergs opted to pursue a natural, herbal treatment when Paul was first diagnosed with squamous cell carcinoma; however, the treatments caused a slew of problems, including painful burns. Now that the squamous cell carcinoma had returned, Paul chose to see a dermatologist, Dr. Robert Hunter in Salt Lake City, and undergo surgery to remove the growing tumor. The surgery was dramatic, but you can hardly tell that Paul nearly lost his face, and his life, to this disease.

Likewise during this time, I had been devoting a significant portion of my time to cancer crusading, often staying up all night, without sleep, working on a wide array of skin cancer-related projects. Recognizing that I was neglecting other aspects of my life, in exchange for Cancer Crusaders, Tiffany shared with me the aforementioned thought: *We must not forget to live.*

Honestly, that has been a difficult lesson for me to learn; a once abstract concept for me to grasp. It has taken me several years to truly understand and accept that while teaching skin cancer prevention is a noble and worthy endeavor, it is not my sole purpose. My personality and the components that comprise the sum of my parts are not synonymously associated with being a "cancer crusader". There exists no indistinguishable line between the two. While, I am deeply passionate about this cause and continue to invest substantial time, talent, effort, energy, resources, and, yes, prayer, toward this cause, I realize that it is not blasphemous to find the balance that lies therein and to admit that I, first and foremost, am a human being; a child of God. Hence, as I serve His children I must not forget to "breathe"—to live. This is what cancer (and the Bergs) has taught me. *We must live.*

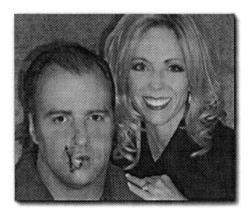

Tiffany Berg pictured with her husband Paul, just after surgery to remove a growing squamous cell carcinoma in his mouth. Paul has been cancer-free since Christmas 2004. *Photo courtesy of the Berg family.*

Utah Melanoma Organizations

The Cancer Crusaders Organization (formerly "Utah Cancer Crusaders")

Mission Statement/Objectives: The mission of The Cancer Crusaders Organization as a registered 501 [c] [3] non-profit service corporation is aimed at providing effective, relevant, and specially tailored skin cancer education to and for our young adult population. Additionally, we are committed to serving as the voice of advocacy; performing compassionate service so as to provide much needed assistance on behalf of the medically-underserved, and to equip individuals with the tools necessary to combat skin cancer. Therefore, our efforts shall be a force for inspiring a more proactive skin cancer prevention stance among the community at-large. Our motto: *"Together we will find a cure for cancer not because we wished for it, but because we worked for it!"®*

Founders (or Directors):
Danielle M. White and Natalie C. Johnson

Point of Contact:
Danielle M. White, President

Full Mailing Address:
P.O. Box 2076
Provo, Utah 84603

Phone:
(801) 863-6351

E-mail Address and Web-site:
info@cancercrusaders.org; www.cancercrusaders.org; www.skincancerribbon.org

---

Are you a 501 [c] [3] non-profit organization & is your status current? Yes

---

Date Founded: 2004

Sources of funding: 50% Fundraising/Membership Dues; 50% Donations

---

Annual Events:
"Only Skin Deep?"® Skin Cancer Prevention Education Conferences throughout national Skin Cancer Awareness Month in May; SunSavvy® Pool Patrol Parties.

On-going Programs:
Developed and host the "ONLY SKIN DEEP?"® Peer Educator's Training and Certification Program; Launched and execute the *"Only Skin Deep?"®* Skin Cancer Prevention Education Campaign to promote the official National Skin Cancer Awareness Symbol®; Implementing the Kaylan's Crusaders Coalition (a sun safety and skin care education program for pageant contestants).

The Cancer Crusaders Organization (formerly "Utah Cancer Crusaders")

Additional Services Provided:
"Conversations With Cancer"®—an award-wining skin cancer prevention education talk show; SunSavvy®—a program that provides sun protection products to melanoma patients of lower income/uninsured households.

Affiliations:
National Coalition for Sun Safety; the National Council on Skin Cancer Prevention; EPA Sun-Wise; the Sun Safety Alliance; "ONE VOICE" for Melanoma; the Utah Cancer Action Network as part of the Utah Cancer Control Program.

Noteworthy Awards/Recognitions:
2005 & 2005 Gold Triangle Award Winners for Excellence in Dermatology Education from the American Academy of Dermatology; Named Utah Valley's 2005 "Angels Among Us."

Misc:
Created and introduced the new, official Skin Cancer Awareness ribbon (a.k.a. National Skin Cancer Symbol©) to American Academy of Dermatology;
Led, in conjunction with the Charlie Guild Melanoma Foundation, legislation for mandatory sun safety education in K-12 public schools throughout Utah (2006);
Led, in conjunction with the Charlie Guild Melanoma foundation, legislation for indoor tanning regulations in Utah (2007).

Utah Cancer Centers

Huntsman Cancer Institute
c/o University of Utah
Atten: Glen M. Bowen, M.D. and Sancy A. Leachman, M.D., Ph.D.
2000 Circle of Hope
Salt Lake City, Utah 84112-5550
Phone: (801) 585-3281; Fax: (801) 581-3389 (fax)

Melanoma Organizations in Other States

Ann's Hope Foundation

Mission Statement/Objectives:
Our mission at Ann's Hope Foundation is to raise awareness of the danger of melanoma cancer and to raise the level of research, early detection, and prevention efforts.

Founders (or Directors):
Ann Harrington and Anne Frentzel

Point of Contact:
Ann Harrington

Full Mailing Address:
P.O. Box 376
Hartland, Wisconsin 53029

Phone:
(262) 305-1350

Web-site:
www.annshope.org

Are you a 501 [c] [3] non-profit organization & is your status current? Yes

Date Founded: 2005

Sources of funding: 100% Donations and Fundraising

Annual Events:
Run/Walk & Gala/Auction.

On-going Programs:
We are only in our second year, so we are still working on developing programs.

The Ashley Fister Cole Foundation

Mission Statement/Objectives:
Our mission at the Ashley Fister Cole Foundation is to "touch a life" through the charitable giving of time, energy, and resources in support of education and healing.

The Ashley Fister Cole Foundation

Founders (or Directors):
Brian S. Cole

Point of Contact:
Brian S. Cole, Executive Director

Full Mailing Address:
9601 Hershour Court
Fairfax, Virginia 22032

Phone:
(703) 323-4683

E-mail Address and Web-site:
bcole2@cox.net; www.ashleyfistercolefoundation.org

Are you a 501 [c] [3] & is your status current? Yes

Date Founded: 2002

Sources of funding: 100% Donations and Fundraising

Annual Events:
"Morning at the Movies" in the Spring; "Driving for Surviving" in the Fall.

On-going Programs:
Semi-annual melanoma education and sun safety newsletter.

Brenda MacDonald Melanoma Foundation

Point of Contact:
Chad MacDonald

Full Mailing Address:
P.O. Box 1600
Sterling, Virginia 20166

Phone:
(703) 480-6600

E-mail Address:
cmacdonald@serviceforceusa.com

Are you a 501 [c] [3] non-profit organization & is your status current? Yes

Colette Coyne Melanoma Awareness Campaign

Mission Statement/Objectives:
The Colette Coyne Melanoma Foundation is dedicated to increasing public awareness regarding the dangers and causes of skin cancer, and changing attitudes and behaviors towards unsafe tanning and sun exposure. We have begun to achieve these goals through the education of parents and children in our schools, public recreational facilities and community-based organizations.

Founders (or Directors):
Colette Coyne

Point of Contact:
Colette Coyne, President

Full Mailing Address:
P.O. Box 1179
New Hyde Park, New York 11040

Phone:
(516) 352-4227

E-mail Address and Web-site:
cmbc1@optonline.net; www.ccmac.org

Are you a 501 [c] [3] non-profit organization & is your status current? Yes

Date Founded: 1998

Sources of funding:
100% Donations and Fundraising

Annual Events:
The foundation sponsors an annual dinner dance and auction, an annual Miles for Melanoma Walk/Run, school based education initiatives and ongoing community education and awareness programs

On-going Programs:
Legislation for tanning bed regulation in New York so as to protect youth from the dangers of tanning.

Additional Services Provided:
Melanoma/Skin Cancer Awareness videos.

Noteworthy Awards/Recognitions:
2002 Gold Triangle Award from the American Academy of Dermatology.

Colette Coyne Melanoma Awareness Campaign

Affiliations:
National Coalition for Sun Safety.

Foreman Foundation (a.k.a. "Knowmelanoma")

Mission Statement/Objectives:
The mission of the Foreman Foundation is to raise funds for medical research that will lead to a cure for melanoma cancer, while heightening awareness as to the causes and symptoms of this disease.

Founders (or Directors):
Phillip Foreman

Point of Contact:
Julianne Rogozewicz, Executive Director

Full Mailing Address:
P.O. BOX 189
Zelienople, Pennsylvania

Phone and Fax:
Phone: (724) 452-9690; Fax: (724) 452-5054

E-mail Address and Web-site:
contact@foremanfoundation.org; www.foremanfoundation.org

Are you a 501 [c] [3] non-profit organization & is your status current? Yes

Date Founded: 1996

Sources of funding:
80% Fundraising; 20% Donations

Annual Events:
Annual Golf Outing; Foreman Foundation Fundraiser Ball and Reverse Drawing; Car Raffle and Art Auction.

Additional Services Provided:
Funding for Research at the Foreman Foundation Melanoma Research Lab;
Education Initiatives on Sun Safety; Corporate Presentations/Outdoor Worker Presentations.

Foreman Foundation (a.k.a. "Knowmelanoma")

Noteworthy Awards/Recognitions:
Along with the Penn State College of Medicine, the Foreman Foundation Melanoma Research Lab at the Penn State Milton S. Hershey Medical Center in Hershey, Pennsylvania, was established in 2002. This lab is making great strides in their therapeutics program. They have received one patent and two provisional patents to date for their research.

Foundation for Melanoma Research

Mission Statement/Objectives:
The Foundation for Melanoma Research is dedicated to raising awareness about melanoma and funding research into increased prevention, early detection, and new treatments.

Founders (or Directors):
Noreen O'Neill

Point of Contact:
Kate O'Neill, President

Full Mailing Address:
3601 Spruce Street
Room 489
Philadelphia, Pennsylvania 19104

Phone and Fax:
Phone: (215) 898-3959; Fax: (215) 898-0980

E-mail Address and Web-site:
info@foundationformelanomaresearch.org; www.foundationformelanomaresearch.org

Are you a 501 [c] [3] non-profit organization & is your status current? Yes

Date Founded: 1999

Annual Events:
Annual "Running for Cover" 5K Run/Walk Fundraiser; Organized first annual Melanoma Research Congress in Philadelphia in June 2003.

Additional Services Provided:
Clark Lecture Series and Melanoma Symposium at the University of Pennsylvania Cancer Center; "Save Our Skin" melanoma awareness/free screening program at Philadelphia-area high schools.

Joanna M. Nicolay Melanoma Foundation

Mission Statement/Objectives:
The mission of the Joanna M. Nicolay Melanoma Foundation is to promote prevention, early detection and research to end melanoma. We will achieve this mission by: Preserving and enhancing our resources; Building relationships; Providing information that can be trusted; Advocating with integrity. By this, the Joanna M. Nicolay Melanoma Foundation will focus on three key objectives: Promote awareness and an understanding of the seriousness of melanoma; Support funding for research to ultimately find a cure for melanoma; Educate the general public on prevention and detection of melanoma.

Founders (or Directors):
Robert E. Nicolay

Point of Contact:
Robert E. Nicolay, Chairman

Full Mailing Address:
P.O. Box 564
Finksburg, Maryland 21048

Phone:
(410) 871-0515

E-mail Address and Web-site:
jmnmf@carr.org; www.melanomaresource.org

Are you a 501 [c] [3] non-profit organization & is your status current? Yes

Date Founded: 2004

Annual Events:
"Melanoma Monday" Press Conference in Maryland (with the Melanoma Research Foundation); SunGuard Man Birthday Contest; Mothers and Others Conference (with the Sun Safety Alliance); Skin Cancer Awareness Fundraising Dinner.

Noteworthy Awards/Recognitions:
Governor of Maryland's "Celebration of Life" Award.

Affiliations:
National Council on Skin Cancer Prevention; Sun Safety Alliance; "ONE VOICE" for Melanoma.

The Kate Verdon Spisak Foundation for Melanoma Awareness and Research, Inc. (a.k.a. "Kate's Foundation")

Mission Statement/Objectives:
The Kate Verdon Spisak Foundation for Melanoma Awareness and Research, Inc. is a not-for-profit organization dedicated to informing the public about melanoma as well as providing financial support to the National Institute of Health's Melanoma Research Program and the patients and families involved in that research.

Founders (or Directors):
The Katie Verdon Spisak Family

Point of Contact:
Renee Strack, Director

Full Mailing Address:
13 Eagle Nest
Colts Neck, New Jersey 07722

Phone:
(732) 772-9876

E-mail Address and Web-site:
www.katesfoundation.com

Are you a 501 [c] [3] non-profit organization & is your status current? Yes

Date Founded: 2000

Annual Events:
A Round for Kate and Kevin: Golf Outing and Silent Auction; Kate's Annual Kick-Off Party Fundraiser.

Additional Services Provided:
Kate's Foundation numerous programs include melanoma awareness campaigns, an educational Web-site, a high school scholarship, free skin cancer screenings, and educational awareness and prevention booths at outdoor sporting events. We distribute free SPF 30 sunscreen, hats, T-shirts and beach towels throughout the year to remind people to always protect their skin from over-exposure to ultraviolet radiation.

Massachusetts Melanoma Foundation

Mission Statement/Objectives:
We, at the Massachusetts Melanoma Foundation, work to save lives from being lost because of melanoma by providing sun awareness education to children in schools throughout the community. We provide support for survivors and their families, and we support research that looks to provide the best tools to change behavior.

Massachusetts Melanoma Foundation

Founders (or Directors):
Deb Girard

Point of Contact:
Deb Girard, Executive Director

Full Mailing Address:
66 Common Wealth
Concord, Massachusetts 01742

Phone and Fax:
Phone: 1-800-557-7632; Fax: (778) 371-0109

E-mail Address and Web-site:
dgirard@massmelanoma.org; www.massmelanoma.org

Are you a 501 [c] [3] non-profit organization & is your status current? Yes

On-going Programs:
Sun Awareness Training Programs for school-based nurses; Winter suns safety (facial scanning and education at ski areas); Melanoma education symposiums for patients and families; Monthly support groups for melanoma patients; Working to pass bed legislation in Massachusetts.

Melanoma Awareness

Mission Statement/Objectives:
Our mission is to raise public awareness of melanoma; provide moral as well as financial support for melanoma victims and their families; support and promote melanoma research.

Founders (or Directors):
Paul Kamman

Point of Contact:
Paul Kamman and Barb Fallstad

Full Mailing Address:
3320 Minnesota Lane
Plymouth, Minnesota 55447

Phone and Fax:
Phone: (763) 544-6210; Fax: (763) 545-1443

Web-site:
www.melanomaawareness.org

Are you a 501 [c] [3] non-profit organization & is your status current? Pending

---

Melanoma Awareness

Date Founded: 2005

Melanoma Education Foundation

Mission Statement/Objectives:
The Melanoma Education Foundation is a non-profit organization devoted to saving lives from melanoma, a common skin cancer that is often deadly unless detected early before there are any symptoms. The Foundation increases awareness of melanoma three ways: Conducts workshops for high school and middle school health educators and provides them with student materials and lesson plans; Provides complete information about early self-detection and prevention of melanoma in a user-friendly Web-site; Conducts talks and facial skin analyzer screenings for area organizations and businesses.

Founders (or Directors):
The Daniel N. Fine Family

Point of Contact:
Stephen A. Fine

Full Mailing Address:
P.O. BOX 2023
Peabody, Massachusetts 01960

Phone and Fax:
Phone: (978) 535-3080; Fax: (978) 535-5602

E-mail Address and Web-site:
MEF@skincheck.org; www.skincheck.org

Are you a 501 [c] [3] non-profit organization & is your status current? Yes

---

Date Founded: 2000

Melanoma Education Foundation

Additional Services Provided:
The MEF conducts numerous community outreach sessions at regional wellness events, public libraries, colleges, city employee sites, and service organizations such as Rotary and Kiwanis Clubs. Talks and facial sun damage screenings are also available to businesses. The MEF seeks to continue and expand high school and middle school educational services, to serve as a resource for health educators in the subject of skin cancer education, and to promote greater public awareness through outreach events. Funding for services is provided primarily by individual contributions, proceeds from special events, and grants from corporations and foundations. Our "Teaching High School Students About Skin Cancer," was developed for health educators. The course, which includes a detailed one-session lesson plan, video, and all required student hand-outs, is registered with the Massachusetts Department of Education, allowing attending teachers to receive credit toward required Professional Development Points. More recently, services were extended to middle schools and to the states of Maine, New Hampshire, Rhode Island, Vermont, Nevada, and New York. By the end of June 2006 the single session SkinCheck® class was mandatory for all entering students in over 400 schools. The program is endorsed by the Massachusetts Interscholastic Athletic Association, and by the Massachusetts Association of Health, Physical Education, Recreation, and Dance.

Melanoma Hope Network

Mission Statement/Objectives:
MHN is a 501 [c] [3] non-profit organization established to bring hope, education and direct personal support to patients diagnosed with melanoma, the most dangerous form of skin cancer. We are especially interested in finding patients affected by the advanced stages of melanoma. We intend to support research; increase patient awareness of clinical trials, and help patients and their primary physicians find the appropriate trials for their particular stage of disease. We also intend to provide a central place for melanoma centers across the country to come to collaborate on data and to update and educate their staff. Above all, we provide hope, help and education to those directly or indirectly affected by melanoma, and support researchers and doctors battling this disease.

Founders (or Directors):
Kent and Jeannie Thornberry with Clay Anderson, MD of the Ellis Fishel Cancer Center

Point of Contact:
Kent Thornberry, Executive Director

Full Mailing Address:
1324 Clarkson/Clayton Center
St. Louis, Missouri 63011

Melanoma Hope Network

Phone and Fax:
Phone: (636) 532-4298; Fax: (636) 530-9960

Email/Web-site
jthornberry@melanomahopenetwork.org; www.melanomahopenetwork.org

Are you a 501 [c] [3] non-profit organization & is your status current? Yes

Date Founded: 2002

Sources of funding:
100% Donations and Fundraising

Annual Events:
Spring Golf Tournament; Fall Dinner/Auction & Trivia Night.

Melanoma Hope Network

Additional Services Provided:
We have the only melanoma-specific web-based clinical trial-finder on the internet. (A patient registers and fills in a short questionnaire about their specific level of disease and the TrialFinder® searches through all trials in our database and tells them what ones they qualify for). It also stores their profit and notifies them as new trials and treatments come available in the future that match their specific profile. Please use the TrialFinder with the understanding that it is **not** a complete listing of all trials/treatments available to you and is not a guarantee that you qualify for any particular trial. You should use this only as one resource in your search for treatment options. You should seek professional advice from your physician or oncologist as to the most appropriate treatment for your specific condition.

1. Additionally, we, at the Melanoma Hope Network, are in the process of recognizing doctors and centers across the country in our Melanoma Hope Network Centers of Excellence program. This program will identify and recognize those doctors and centers across the country that offer the full treatment and support melanoma patients need while battling this disease. This way, patients can quickly resource that across the country treats the most melanoma patients.

2. Center must have multiple disciplines under one roof or working agreements between collaborating groups that provide patient with seamless care in dermatology, surgery (general or surgical oncology), medical oncology, and radiation oncology.

3. Center must have at least two melanoma specific clinical trials actively recruiting.

4. Center should be able to provide a doctor and nurse or office staff person as a MHN contact person/team leader for referrals and other information needs.

5. Center must provide a short paragraph that describes the support services that are available to their patients and their families. These services may be provided directly by the center or via collaborative arrangements with other support agencies.

6. Center must provide a short paragraph that describes how this center participates in community education.

Melanoma International Foundation

Mission Statement/Objectives:
Our mission at MIF is to save lives now from melanoma by providing hope and empowering with education.

Founders (or Directors):
Catherine M. Poole

Melanoma International Foundation

Point of Contact:
Catherine M. Poole, President

Full Mailing Address:
250 Mapleflower Road
Glenmoore, Pennsylvania 19343

Phone:
(610) 942-3432

E-mail Address and Web-site:
info@melanomaintl.org; www.melanomaintl.org

Are you a 501 [c] [3] non-profit organization & is your status current? Yes

Annual Events:
"Safe From the Sun" in Philadelphia, Pennsylvania, Seattle, Washington, and Phoenix, Arizona.

On-going Programs:
A 24-hour international patient and caregiver support hotline.

Additional Services Provided:
We teach skin self-examination and sun safety to the public in all venues is so as to have an even greater impact on mortality rates. We can companies, during our Lunchtime Learning Program, how to properly perform a thorough self-skin examination in just two minutes.

Noteworthy Awards/Recognitions:
Our Web-site recently received the Oncolink Editor's Choice Award. Our founder, Catherine Poole, was also named 2006 "Advocate of the Year" by The Cancer Crusaders Organization and SunSavvy, LLC.

Affiliations:
We are a participating member in: C-Change, formally The National Dialogue on Cancer; the American Association For Cancer Research; the National Council For Skin Cancer Prevention; the American Academy of Dermatology's National Coalition for Sun Safety; the American Society of Clinical Oncology; the Pennsylvania Governor's Cancer Advisory Board; the National Cancer Institute's (NCI) Cancer Advocates in Research and Related Activities; "ONE VOICE" for Melanoma.

Melanoma Research Foundation

Mission Statement/Objectives:
The mission of the Melanoma Research Foundation is to support medical research for finding effective treatments and eventually a cure for melanoma; To educate patients and physicians about the prevention, diagnosis and treatment of melanoma; To act as an advocate for the melanoma community to raise the awareness of this disease and the need for a cure.

Founders (or Directors):
Diana Ashby

Point of Contact:
Linda Pilkington, Executive Director

Full Mailing Address:
24 Old Georgetown Road,
Princeton, New Jersey 08540

Phone:
1-800-MRF-1290

E-mail Address and Web-site:
Linda@melanoma.org; www.melanoma.org; www.mpip.org

Are you a 501 [c] [3] non-profit organization & is your status current? Yes

Date Founded: 1996

Sources of funding:
33%; Donations and Membership; 56% Fundraising and Events; 11% Grants

Annual Events:
Wings of Hope Dinner in New York; Don Aranow Golf Tournament in New York; HackNS-mack Celebrity Golf Tournament in California; Other annual local grass roots events.

On-going Programs:
Major research grants for basic and translational research reviewed by leading researchers according to the National Cancer Institute (NCI) standards and key opinion leaders on our Scientific Advisory Committee; the National Patient Symposiums; the Miles for Melanoma Program.

Additional Services Provided:
Patient and caregiver support and education via the Melanoma Patient Information Page (www.mpip.org) and our toll-free number; Assistance with grass roots events and activities.

Melanoma Research Foundation

Noteworthy Awards/Recognitions:
The MRF was instrumental in organizing the first "ONE VOICE" for Melanoma meeting in March 2006 which brought together all melanoma-specific foundations. The MRF also was instrumental in forming the Society of Melanoma Researchers, now a very active organization of researchers.

Melanoma Support & Education Foundation

Mission Statement/Objectives:
We, at the Melanoma Support & Education Foundation, are a 501[c] [3] non-profit foundation created to provide support and education to the melanoma community, inform the public on the prevention of melanoma and promote sun safe habits.

Founders (or Directors):
Staci Vazquez

Point of Contact:
Staci Vazquez or Robin Petry

Full Mailing Address:
310 Clay Street
Ottawa, Illinois 61350

Phone and Fax:
(815) 212-4924 (phone)

E-mail Address and Web-site:
Staci@melanomasupport.org; www.melanomasupport.org

Are you a 501 [c] [3] non-profit organization & is your status current? Yes

Date Founded: 2005

Sources of funding:
100% Donations and Fundraising

Annual Events:
5K run in Ottawa, Illinois (May); Golf Tournament in Houston, Texas (September); Melanoma Monday (in connection with the AAD) in Chicago, Illinois (May).

On-going Programs:
Awareness/Education on Sun Safety

Additional Services Provided:
Support Baskets to melanoma patients; Sun Safety information to Youth Sports Camp participants.

Mollie Biggane Melanoma Foundation

Mission Statement/Objectives:
Increase awareness for melanoma prevention, provide information and services on skin cancer detection, and support melanoma patients through education of the latest treatments. Our goals are: To implement our skin cancer awareness program in every High School/Middle School Health class curriculum; To raise awareness through sun protection programs and mole identification techniques; To help existing patients and families of patients to understand the latest technologies available and how to navigate their way to the best solution.

Founders (or Directors):
The Mollie Biggane Family

Point of Contact:
Jack Biggane, Executive Director

Full Mailing Address:
168 Euston Road
Garden City, New York 11530

Phone and Fax
Phone: (516) 741-2056; Fax: (516) 877-2537

E-mail Address and Web-site
bigganej@optonline.net; www.molliesfund.org

Are you a 501 [c] [3] & is your status current? Yes

Date Founded: 2000

Sources of funding:
100% Donations and Fundraising

Annual Events:
Annual September Golf Outing, Annual Mollie's Fundraising Dinner and Auction.

Mollie Biggane Melanoma Foundation

On-going Programs:
Produced educational skin cancer DVD, "The Dark Side of the Sun", our goal is to have it distributed through health departments in NY schools within the year. The DVD has been accepted into an existing Skin Cancer Curriculum in Massachusetts and we are anticipating acceptance into a program in the Maine schools; Contacted the 11 zone presidents of the New York State Association of Health, Physical Education, Recreation and Dance and offered to present at their annual meetings; Met with the Assistant Superintendent of the Garden City school district to solicit help for our health class agenda; National advertising campaigns on Sun Safety and Skin Cancer Awareness; Created an educational wallet sized self skin-exam brochure and sent over 5,000 to colleges and universities throughout the U.S; Participated in the Hofstra University Wellness Fair in August 2006 where we distributed educational materials and other resources to staff members in preparation for their interaction with incoming students; On-going involvement in health awareness days on college campuses across the country, supplying them with educational materials and sunscreen.

Additional Services Provided:
Distribution of hats, sunscreen and educational materials; free full-body skin screenings; melanoma treatment symposiums; health fairs.

Outrun the Sun, Inc.

Mission Statement/Objectives:
Our mission is to increase awareness of the risk factors for melanoma and other skin cancers and to raise funds for medical research leading to new treatments and cures for melanoma.

Founders (or Directors):
Anita Day, Jonna MacDougall, Jennifer Patton, and Marci Reddick

Point of Contact:
Anita Day, President

Full Mailing Address:
9202 Briarclift Road
Indianapolis, Indiana 46256

E-mail Address and Web-site:
anita@outrunthesun.org; www.outrunthesun.org

Are you a 501 [c] [3] non-profit organization & is your status current? Yes

Date Founded: 2002

Sources of funding:
100% Donations and Fundraising

Outrun the Sun, Inc.

Annual Events:
"Out Run the Sun" 5K Fundraising/Skin Cancer Awareness Run in Indiana.

On-going Programs:
Monthly Melanoma Networking Support Group at the Wellness Community of Central Indiana.

Additional Services Provided:
Education and Outreach.

Sabra Daly Rightmire Foundation for Metastic Melanoma Education and Research (also known as "BeSunSensible")

Mission Statement/Objectives:
BeSunSensible is a 501 [c] [3] non-profit organization established in April 2000 as The Sabra Dalby Rightmire Foundation for Melanoma Education and Research by the friends and family of Sabra Dalby Rightmire, an exceptional woman who died at the age of 27 after a 10 month long battle with melanoma, the most lethal form of skin cancer. BeSunSensible's mission is to prevent melanoma through educational initiatives targeted at parents and caregivers of young children by educating them on:

- The dangers of sun exposure

- The lifelong need for comprehensive sun protection.

- The disease of skin cancer/melanoma

E-mail Address and Web-site:
Jde1130@yahoo.com; www.besunsensible.org

Are you a 501 [c] [3] non-profit organization & is your status current? Yes

Date Founded: 2000

The Sidney J. Malawer Memorial Foundation

Mission Statement/Objectives:
Our mission is to educate the public on ways to prevent skin cancer and promote the importance of early detection through frequent skin screenings. Through this education, we hope to change public attitudes and behaviors toward sun exposure, teach people how to properly protect themselves, and lower the toll from this devastating disease. In coordination with Suburban Hospital Healthcare Systems, we have developed community outreach programs and eventually hope to help Suburban develop a Department of Excellence in dermatological oncology.

Founders: Leslie Malawer Keenan, Carol Malawer, and Judith Malawer Walker

The Sidney J. Malawer Memorial Foundation

Point of Contact: Leslie Malawer Keenan

Full Mailing Address:
12305 Riding Fields Road
Rockville, Maryland 20850.

Phone and Fax:
Phone: (301) 977-2366; Fax: (301) 417-9635

Email and Web-site:
info@blockitout.org; www.blockitout.org

Are you a 501 [c] [3] non-profit organization & is your status current? Yes

Date Founded: 2002

Annual Events:
The Sidney J. Malawer Memorial Golf Classic and Dinner Fundraiser.

On-going Programs:
Skin cancer screenings; Sun Safety poster contests for elementary/middle school students.

Additional Services Provided:
Donate funds to the Suburban Cancer Hospital Programs; write and implement Sun Safety initiatives; distribute sun safety tool kits and interactive learning programs for elementary/middle schools.

Skin Cancer Awareness Foundation

Mission Statement/Objectives:
This is a 501[c[[3] non-profit organization whose purpose is to increase awareness, stress education and urge prevention of skin cancer by changing attitudes, behaviors and environments to promote sun safety. Educational materials are available to provide to schools and other youth-based organizations at no charge, which focuses sun safety education and skin cancer prevention for children in athletic groups and their parents. Fundraising is done through special family events to raise money for youth-based sports organizations, the Skin Cancer Awareness Foundation, and elementary school sun safety education programs.

Point of Contact:
Bill Barth and Ann Haas, M.D.

Full Mailing Address:
2685 Billy's Road
Minden, Nevada 89423

Phone and Fax:
Phone: 1-877-478-6227; Fax: (775) 267-4318

Skin Cancer Awareness Foundation

E-mail Address and Web-site:
info@skincaf.org; www.skincaf.org; www.kidscoolschoolprogram.org

On-going Programs:
Sun Safe Youth Sports Program. This program was developed to work with youth sports groups to educate and eliminate skin cancer among youth athletes. Sun safety information is made available at a variety of youth sports events which will create awareness of sun safe behavior; Sun Smart Kids Cool School Program. This is a collaborative venture between two 501 [c] [3] non profit organizations with an interest in sun safety education for children. The Sun Safe City Program of Davis, California combined resources with the Skin Cancer Awareness Foundation to create the "Kids Cool School Program". This is an age-appropriate presentation which can be given by a volunteer medical professional/school nurse in the classroom or small assembly format. The Program has a color book with accompanying PowerPoint presentation K-3 graders, and the same type of materials (more advanced) for use in grades 4-8. The program also comes with suggestions on presentation and implementation of the teaching program. This was created for volunteers who had the interest in presenting this material in a fun, age-appropriate manner, but lacked the materials to take into the classroom. The Program was reviewed by dermatologists and teachers, prior to initial implementation. The Program is available for downloading, upon request.

Sun Protection Foundation (a.k.a. The Children's Melanoma Prevention Foundation)

Mission Statement/Objectives:
To increase a student's knowledge of the risks associated with unprotected sun exposure; To improve sun protection behaviors; To de-trivialize skin cancer; To educate health care professionals about skin cancer prevention and early detection; To prevent death due to skin cancer.

Founders (or Directors):
Maryellen Maguire-Eisen RN, MSN, CS, OCN

Point of Contact:
Maryellen Maguire-Eisen

Full Mailing Address:
P.O. Box 254
Hingham, Massachusetts 02043

Phone:
(781) 875-1773

Web-site:
www.melanomaprevention.org

Are you a 501 [c] [3] non-profit organization & is your status current? Yes

Sun Protection Foundation (a.k.a. The Children's Melanoma Prevention Foundation)

Date Founded: 2003

Sources of funding:
70% Donations, 20% Grants, 10% Fundraising

Annual Events:
Skin Cancer Workshops for nurses and health Educators both nationally and locally

On-going Programs:
Learn-Not-2-Burn Program

Additional Services Provided:
Patient counseling; a UV Monitoring Program; support, research, and professional publications.

Noteworthy Awards/Recognitions:
2002 Neutrogena Corporation Community Service Award; 2005 Dermatology Nurses Association Research Award.

Affiliations:
Dana Farber Cancer Institute; Boston University; Dermatology Nurses Association; Women's Dermatology Society.

Susan Fazio Foundation for Melanoma Research

Mission Statement/Objectives:
The mission of the Susan Fazio Foundation for Melanoma Research is to raise funds to support research and increase awareness of Metastatic Melanoma and Mucosal Melanoma cancers.

Founders (or Directors):
Joe Fazio, Chris Fazio, Michael Fazio, and Cara Fazio Mundell

Point of Contact:
Cara Fazio Mundell

Full Mailing Address
685 Misty Hollow Drive
Maple Glen, Pennsylvania 19002

Phone:
(267) 251-4585

E-mail Address and Web-site:
cara@susanfazio.org; www.susanfazio.org

Are you a 501 [c] [3] & is your status current? Yes

Susan Fazio Foundation for Melanoma Research

Date Founded: 2006

Sources of funding:
100% Donations and Fundraising

Annual Events:
Fall Silent Auction and Dinner; Spring Happy Hour Fundraiser.

Additional Services Provided:
Fundraising for the Melanoma Research Foundation.

Teb's Troops, Inc.

Mission Statement/Objectives:
Teb's Troops is a not-for-profit organization started in honor of Tricia E. Black, ("Teb"), was diagnosed with stage IV metastatic melanoma. Wanting to rally her "troops" during her war with cancer and desiring to make something positive come from the negative, Teb asked her friends to help her design and sell a bracelet, the profits of which would go to organizations that support the treatment, prevention, and research of melanoma. (Teb passed away in 2006 at the age of 29).

Founders (or Directors):
The Tricia E. Black Family

Point of Contact:
Sarah Fischer, President

Full Mailing Address:
Teb's Troops, Inc.
5859 N Winthrop Avenue #3
Chicago, Illinois 60660

E-mail Address and Web-site:
sarah@tebstroops.org; www.tebstroops.org

Are you a 501 [c] [3] non-profit organization & is your status current? Yes

Date Founded: 2006

Sources of funding:
100% Donations and Fundraising

Annual Events:
"A Call to Arms" Teb's Troops Annual Fundraising Event

Tech Sgt. Alan "Al" C. Lawson Melanoma Cancer Foundation (a.k.a. The Lawson Cancer Foundation)

Mission Statement/Objectives:
"Save A Life: Protect Your Birthday Suit"

Founders (or Directors):
Lori Spicer-Lawson

Point of Contact:
Lori Spicer-Lawson

Full Mailing Address:
Tech. Sgt. Alan "Al" C. Lawson Melanoma Cancer Foundation
1222 Koufax Drive
Chatham, Illinois 62629

E-mail Address and Web-site:
loriespicer@aol.com; www.2-pay-it-forward.com

Are you a 501 [c] [3] non-profit organization & is your status current? Yes

Date Founded: 2003

On-going Programs:
Young Heroes.

Tiffany Weirbach Melanoma Foundation

Mission Statement/Objectives:
To aggressively inform and educate on the serious dangers of Malignant Melanoma and other skin cancers; To promote self-skin examinations, proper physician screening, early detection, treatment options, prevention; To provide financial assistance (as funds are available) to those suffering from malignant melanoma; To work towards the eradication of this disease that kills thousands each year; To share knowledge and information we have gained from the courageous fight of our 24-year-old daughter who, at age 21 was diagnosed with malignant melanoma, was taken by this disease on October 8, 2001; To provide information to patients looking for financial assistance, treatments, treatment centers and options as well as educate on prevention by the use of sunscreens and early detection.

Founders (or Directors):
The Tiffany Weirbach Family

Point of Contact:
Judd Weirbach

Tiffany Weirbach Melanoma Foundation

Full Mailing Address:
P.O. BOX 1386
Redmond, Oregon 97756

E-mail and Web-site:
judd@dadsgirl.org; www.tiffanysmelanomafoundation.org

Are you a 501 [c] [3] non-profit organization & is your status current? Yes

Date Founded: 2001

Sources of funding:
100% Donations

Noteworthy Awards/Recognitions:
Recently published nationally acclaimed book entitled Dad's Girl that is available at www.dadsgirl.org

Timothy Aycock Melanoma Research Organization

Mission Statement/Objectives:
Our mission is to continue his heroic battle against melanoma by increasing awareness about this lethal disease, contributing to cutting-edge medical research, and providing information to those who struggle with melanoma's devastating effects.

Founders (and Directors):
Jonathan Aycock

Point of Contact:
Jonathan Aycock, Executive Director

Full Mailing Address:
P.O. Box 1741
Leesburg, Virginia 20177

Phone:
(703) 484-5826

E-mail and Web-site:
jaycock@cisco.com; www.melanomafund.org

Are you a 501 [c] [3] non-profit organization & is your status current? Yes

Date Founded: 2003

Sources of funding: 100% Donations

National Skin Cancer Organizations

American Academy of Dermatology

Mission Statement/Objectives:
The American Academy of Dermatology is the largest, most influential, and most representative of all dermatologic associations. With a membership of more than 15,000 physicians worldwide, the Academy is committed to: 1) advancing the diagnosis and medical, surgical and cosmetic treatment of the skin, hair and nails; 2) advocating high standards in clinical practice, education, and research in dermatology; and 3) supporting and enhancing patient care for a lifetime of healthier skin, hair and nails.

Founders (or Directors):
Ronald A. Henrichs, CAE, Executive Director and CEO; 2006/2007 President: Stephen P. Stone, M.D.

Point of Contact:
Communications Department

Full Mailing Address:
930 E. Woodfield Road
Schaumburg, Illinois 0173

Phone and Fax:
Phone: (847) 330-0230 (phone); Fax: (847) 330-8907

Web-site:
www.aad.org

Are you a 501 [c] [3] non-profit organization & is your status current? Yes

Date Founded: 1938

Sources of funding:
29% Meetings Revenue; 24% Membership Dues; 19% Grants and Contributions; 23% Publication Royalties; 5% Other.

Annual Events:
Melanoma Monday Conference (first Monday in May); National Melanoma/Skin Cancer Detection and Prevention Month (May).

American Academy of Dermatology

On-going Programs:
On behalf of Skin Cancer Reduction: Intervention Plan for Tomorrow (S.C.R.I.P.T.): National Melanoma/Skin Cancer Screening program; Shade Structure Grant program; Play Smart When It Comes to the Sun™ (baseball skin cancer screening program); Make Sun Safety Your Goal™ (soccer skin cancer awareness program); skin cancer public service announcements; core member of the National Council on Skin Cancer Prevention; host of National Coalition for Sun Safety.

Other Services You Provide:
Public education materials (pamphlets) on more than 65 dermatologic conditions; dedicated Web site to provide the public with detailed information regarding seven dermatologic conditions, including skin cancer.

Noteworthy Awards/Recognitions:
Publicity Club of Chicago Golden Trumpet Award for Skin Cancer Awareness Activities; Public Relations Society of America Bronze Anvil Award of Commendation; Expect to receive a Guinness World Record for the most skin cancer screenings performed in a single day.

National Council on Skin Cancer Prevention

Mission Statement/Objectives:
The National Council on Skin Cancer Prevention facilitates skin cancer awareness, prevention, and early detection through education and promotion of sun safe behaviors. Together we will reduce the mortality and suffering from this devastating disease. Our goals are as follows: To coordinate a public health response to nationwide efforts to reduce skin cancer incidence, morbidity and mortality, including sharing research findings, planning joint programs and conferences, and targeting audience-specific initiatives; To raise the importance of skin cancer prevention and support prevention initiatives on the agendas of relevant national, state, and local organizations; To develop and support partnerships to extend and reinforce core recommendations and encourage behavior change; To increase awareness and prevention behaviors among all populations, with special programs addressing high-risk populations (including children, young adults, outdoor workers, and athletes) through education to health professionals, parents, teachers, and the public.

Founders (or Directors):
Allan Halpern, MD and Alan Geller, RN, MPH

Point of Contact:
Michelle Baker

Full Mailing Address:
5800 Wilson Lane
Bethesda, Maryland 20817

National Council on Skin Cancer Prevention

Phone:
(301) 529-2031

E-mail Address and Web-site:
www.skincancerprevention.org

Are you a 501 [c] [3] non-profit organization & is your status current? Yes

Date Founded: 1998

Sources of funding:
100% membership dues and donations from members

Annual Events:
Bi-annual meetings.

On-going Programs:
Conferences and Symposiums on skin cancer issues.

The Skin Cancer Foundation

Mission Statement/Objectives:
To reduce the incidence of skin cancer through the promotion of prevention, early detection, and effective treatment. Our goals are as follows: To control the epidemic; To prevent skin cancers through public education campaigns about the need for sun protection all year around from birth to old age; To change public attitudes towards tanning and sun exposure to encourage detection of skin cancers at the earliest stage when they are almost always curable; To improve skin cancer care by offering physician education and training programs; To support research into new diagnostic techniques and therapies; To focus attention on melanoma, the most life-threatening of the skin cancers; To teach children and their caregivers about the importance of developing appropriate sun protection behavior early in life; To stimulate public education programs abroad. The Skin Cancer Foundation achieves its mission through nationwide public and professional education programs aimed at increasing:

- Public awareness
- Sun protection and sun safety
- Skin self-examination
- Melanoma understanding
- Continuing medical education
- International action

The Skin Cancer Foundation

Founders (or Directors):
Dr. Perry Robbins, President

Full Mailing Address:
149 Madison Avenue # 901
New York, New York 10016

Phone:
1-800-SKIN-490

E-mail Address and Web-site:
info@skincancer.org; www.skincancer.org

Are you a 501 [c] [3] non-profit organization & is your status current? Yes

Date Founded: 1979

Annual Events:
International World Conference on Cancers of the Skin (2007 conference will be held in Amsterdam in June).

Sun Safety Alliance

Mission Statement/Objectives:
To build awareness of the dangers of over exposure to UV radiation as a cause of skin cancer and to promote public understanding via education and activities hat will lead to change in personal behavior and adoption of sun safe practices while enjoying the benefits of outdoor activity.

Founders (or Directors):
The National Association of Chain Drug Stores

Point of Contact:
Phillip L. Schneider, President

Full Mailing Address:
413 N. Lee Street
Alexandria, Virginia 22314

Phone:
(703) 837-4202

E-mail Address and Web-site:
pschneider@sunsafetyalliance.org; www.sunsafetyalliance.org

Are you a 501 [c] [3] non-profit organization & is your status current? Yes

Sun Safety Alliance

Date Founded: 2004

Sources of funding:
100% donations

Annual Events:
Sun Safety Week, declared by Congress as the first full week of June.

On-going Programs:
Mothers and Others Against Skin Cancer, "Learn, Don't Burn" program, and other related activities.

Other Services You Provide:
Public speaking

Noteworthy Awards/Recognitions:
2006 Gold Triangle Award from the American Academy of Dermatology; "Outstanding Public Awareness Campaign" from the Pubic Relations Society of American; Social Responsibility Award from Women in Public Relations; national coverage three times on the *Today* show, Recognition from the US Surgeon General's Office for public education.

Affiliations:
National Council on Skin Cancer Prevention.

United States Environmental Protection Agency's SunWise Program

Mission Statement/Objectives:
The SunWise Program will raise public awareness of ozone depletion and potential health effects from overexposure to ultraviolet radiation to achieve sustained sun-safe behavior. The goal of the SunWise Program is to reduce the incidence of skin cancer by changing attitudes and behavior concerning sun exposure. The SunWise Program's objectives are as follows: To reduce overexposure to UV radiation by fostering awareness of its associated health risks and teaching simple steps to avoid over-exposure; To improve the delivery, usefulness, and availability of accurate and timely UV Index data to the public to improve their day-to-day decision making regarding sun safety; To build capacity in communities to ensure that SunWise becomes self-sustaining and used independently.

Founders (or Directors):
Drusilla Hufford and Linda Rutsch

Point of Contact:
Linda Rutsch

United States Environmental Protection Agency's SunWise Program

Full Mailing Address:
1200 Pennsylvania Avenue
NW Mailcode 6205 J
Washington, D.C., 20460

Phone and Fax:
Phone: (202) 343-9924; Fax: (202) 343-2338

E-mail and Web-site:
sunwise@epa.gov; www.epa.gov/sunwise

Are you a 501 [c] [3] non-profit organization & is your status current? No. We are a government agency and therefore are federally funded.

Date Founded: 1998

Sources of funding:
100% federal appropriations

On-going Programs:
The SunWise Program is an environmental and health education program that aims to teach children and their caregivers how to protect themselves from overexposure to the sun. Schools and other non-profit organizations that register receive, free of charge, a SunWise Tool Kit with over 40 standards based, cross-curricular activities for grades K-8; a UV sensitive Frisbee for hands-on experiments and fun; story and activity books; poster; video; policy guidance, and more.

Other Services You Provide:
Print brochures and booklets on ultraviolet radiation (UV), ozone depletion, environmental health effects, and sun safety are available at no cost by contacting SunWise at sunwise@epa.gov. An electronic library of these materials is also available on the SunWise Web-site. The SunWise Web site also has interactive games for children and additional educational resources such as introductory presentations and videos. SunWise also provides the UV Index, a forecast of UV intensity for your community, at: www.epa.gov/sunwise/uvindex.html. EPA will issue a UV Alert if the level of solar UV radiation is predicted to be unusually high. The public may sign up to have the UV Index or UV Alert delivered to their e-mail address at: https://enviroflash.epa.gov/uv/Subscriber.do?method=start

Noteworthy Awards/Recognitions:
1999 Excellence in Education Award by the American Academy of Dermatology; the Federal Council on Skin Cancer Prevention's Annual Achievement Award in 2002; the Excellence in Cancer Awareness Award in 2003 by the Congressional Families Action for Cancer Awareness Program of the Cancer Research and Prevention Foundation; the OncoLink award in 2004 for excellence in Web-site information on cancer; the SHADE Foundation's Golden Glove award in 2004.

Additional Resources

In addition to the melanoma organizations listed, there various books that have been written about melanoma skin cancer that are worthy of mention and are useful as you pursue your research. A few of those books include the following:

- 100 Questions and Answers about Melanoma & Other Skin Cancers by Edward F. McClay
- Dad's Girl by Judd Weirbach
- The Melanoma Book: A Complete Guide to Prevention and Treatment, Including the Early Detection Self-Exam Body Map by Howard L. Kaufman
- Melanoma: Prevention, Detection, and Treatment by Catherine M. Poole and DuPont Guerry
- Saving Your Skin: Prevention, Early Detection, and Treatment of Melanoma and other Skin Cancers by Dr. Barney Kenet and Patricia Lawler
- Sun Protection for Life by Mary Mills Barrow and John F. Barrow
- What You Really Need to Know about Moles and Melanoma (A Johns Hopkins Press Health Book) by Jill R. Schofield

PART IV

Perspectives on Skin Cancer

A) Young Adults

- Natalie Johnson

- Kaylan Judd

B) Parents

- Colette Coyne

- Valerie Guild

C) A Survivor

- Robin Lawrence

Perspectives on Skin Cancer: Natalie Johnson

Interview conducted on July 22, 2005

The fourth child of six, 27-year-old Natalie Johnson was raised in Bountiful, Utah and graduated, with honors, from Brigham Young University in 2002 with a degree in Accounting. A week after graduation, Natalie captured the title of Miss Utah where she served for a solid year promoting "Skin Cancer Prevention Education" as her platform.

As mentioned earlier in this book, I had the privilege of meeting Natalie when she was serving as Miss Utah 2002-2003. Our first official face-to-face meeting was on January 28, 2003. I was organizing and hosting a skin cancer prevention education conference and survivor's luncheon at Utah Valley State College. Natalie was the special keynote speaker at this event, where she spoke to students about the importance of sun safety. We immediately began working together on behalf of the skin cancer community. During a span of six months, Natalie and I teamed up countless times to collaborate on various projects and, from thereon, we were to become good, close friends. In my life, I have encountered a slew of incredible people—people who have touched me and inspired me to varying degrees. Natalie, however, is an abundantly talented human being, who never ceases to amaze me.

Arguably the one individual who has truly pioneered the skin cancer crusade; she initiated a real grassroots movement and has inspired people, particularly young adults, to become actively engaged in the cause. She is a person I hold in high regard and great esteem. It has been, and continues to be, a privilege to be associated with Natalie. She is a young woman of great integrity and intelligence, and one who demonstrates a continuing compassion and sensitivity for those touched by this disease. When she enters a room, or steps up to a podium to speak, she commands an audience. People respond to Natalie. They relate to her. They respond to her. Natalie has much to share with the skin cancer community. She is a person I respect and admire as a peer, a colleague, and as a friend.

On becoming involved:

"We [my family and I] were generally aware of the risks. Several of my siblings and I have had suspicious moles removed. None of them were melanoma, but they were all dysplastic, which means they were on their way to becoming a skin cancer. Then, several years later, our general awareness turned into an acute sensitivity when my older brother, Eric, who was just 21-years-old at the time was diagnosed with malignant melanoma—the deadliest form of skin cancer. My brother was diagnosed with the disease [...] after just two months of receiving chemotherapy treatments he, unfortunately, passed away. That was May 8, 1999.And so ever since then, I have launched myself into this 'crusade', if you will, against skin cancer because the more I researched this disease, the more I learned how preventable it was, which, to me, is such an interesting message; it's preventable; it's a message of hope. Often times, I think, we hear the word cancer and think it is synonymous with the word death, but in the case of skin cancer, it doesn't have to be that way because 95% of skin cancers are attributed to over-exposure to ultraviolet radiation and that's completely preventable. The main source of that comes from the sun. So as long as we take those precautions we can do ourselves a great favor and dramatically decrease our risk for getting this deadly disease."

On losing her older brother, Eric:

"I never realized how much of a problem skin cancer was until after my brother's diagnosis [...] Most people don't realize that too much sun exposure is the most preventable cause of melanoma. If you catch suspicious moles and sun-spots, which may be precursors to cancer early enough, you can prevent them from becoming cancerous."

On creating a prevention mind-set among youth:

"As far as prevention goes, it is important to keep in mind, again, is that skin cancer is caused, overwhelmingly by over-exposure to ultraviolet radiation. So, you need to protect yourself from the sun. I know it is hard to do. In general, as a society, we like to be outside [...] and I'm one of those people, you just have to be smart about it."

On fighting the culture of tan:

"It is very difficult to change people's mindset. Right now, if you were to go up to anyone on the street and ask them if they looked if they looked healthier with a tan they would most likely say 'yes' but we know now that any type of tan on your skin, no matter the degree of darkness, is a sign of damage. And so it is hard for people to understand that the sun damage they are incurring right now will affect them years down the road, and not only is there that heightened risk for skin cancer, but also, tanning can cause other damage to skin such as permanent loss of elasticity, age spots, premature wrinkles. So there are image conscious things to consider when tanning and out in the sun. So, it is a difficult mindset to combat especially since a lot of people in Hollywood do promote more of that tan look. So, to kind of bridge that gap between the day when people start to see a tan as unhealthy, we do have the use of self-tanning lotions. And I do think they have come along way in last few years from turning you orange to varying shades of brown, with occasional streaking. That is something I advocate the use of if people still want to achieve that tan look. It is difficult to change that mindset overnight, but I guess the bottom-line comes down to this: if you are tanning to look healthier it is ultimately self-defeating. It does increase your risk for skin cancer, and then there are other considerations as far as how it affects your looks later on in life. So, you're sacrificing your health in the future to quote 'look better' today, which, to me, doesn't make much sense. People have to know that what they're doing right now has permanent consequences. Once you've sustained that damage to your skin, there's no cream, no laser surgery; there's nothing that can reverse that damage."

On being a former Miss Utah:

"As a former Miss Utah, Natalie has been able to make a positive impact in spreading knowledge about this deadly but often ignored disease," says Mike Johnson, Natalie's younger brother. "I've been able to go with Natalie places and see what happens, what melanoma is and see how people really do suffer. She was even invited to speak at the American Academy of Dermatology [2005 Melanoma Monday Press Conference in New York City]." Natalie's response: "I am so fortunate to be able to honor Eric's memory."*

Natalie's contributions to the cause:

Prior to co-founding The Cancer Crusaders Organization, and even before introducing the new, official National Skin Cancer Awareness Symbol© to the American Academy of Dermatology (and to the world), Natalie was instrumental in securing more than $4 million from the Utah State Legislature for melanoma research at Huntsman Cancer Institute where she worked in the high-risk melanoma unit as a mole mapping technician. Natalie, over a span of seven years, has taught more than 500,000 Utahns, has appeared on and in a plethora of media outlets, including <u>SHAPE Magazine</u> (May 2006 edition), has spoken at dermatology conventions, and continues to inspire other young adults to become involved with the skin cancer community. Above all, through the introduction of a national Skin Cancer Awareness ribbon, Natalie was single-handedly paved the way for a tremendous influx of vital skin cancer prevention work to be developed and, in turn, dramatically increase the level of awareness for this common, yet preventable disease.

> "There needed to be a symbol that stands for all the types of skin cancer and that can bring a little bit more hope than a black ribbon. It [the ribbon] represents the cause of skin cancer (overexposure to ultraviolet light) as well as serving as a message of hope."

Natalie's message:

"As college students and young adults, we sometimes think that we're invincible or that cancer is an older person's disease. I want to tell people that this is a disease that can affect anyone, no matter the age."

Perspectives on Skin Cancer: Kaylan Judd

Interview conducted on March 16, 2006

As the oldest child of five, Kaylan is consistently setting an example for her friends and family to follow by diligently practicing year-round sun safety. And at age 16, she is an impressive young woman who rekindles my hope for raising a prevention-minded generation of youth that not only recognizes the importance of protecting themselves from skin cancer, but actively serves the community by teaching others about skin cancer prevention. I have worked with Kaylan in various capacities, watching her adopt "Skin Cancer Awareness" as her platform for the Miss Teen Utah International competition. I marvel that, in her spare time when she could be hanging out the mall with other teenagers, Kaylan is traveling to local elementary schools throughout Utah using the Environmental Protection Agency's SunWise program and teaching them about good sun safety habits. This should come as no surprise to me. After all, she is the daughter of Tiffany Berg, one of my mentors, and "the apple does not fall far from the tree."

On becoming involved:

"The personal reasons why I got involved were because my dad went though it. He was diagnosed with skin cancer three years ago and went through two bouts of it. We thought it had gone away the first time, but it had come back and he has lost quite a bit of his face because of it. Now, he won't ever be able to use a straw or whistle, but at least he is still here."

On watching her stepfather, Paul, battle skin cancer:

"It was scary," said Kaylan's eight-year-old sister, Hannah. Kaylan agreed. "It was hard for us to watch him go through that; to go through treatments, to go through surgery and to see him lose part of his face. It was scary, especially when you think that it happened twice."

On creating a prevention mind-set among youth:

"First of all, people, especially my age, need to realize that every blistering sunburn you get before you're 18, it increases your risk by at least 60%. I tell [my peers] that can you get burned faster skiing down the mountains then standing on the beach in Los Angeles, and people are just shocked. They are shocked about how easy it is to get skin cancer, and also how easy it is to prevent it. If they just think, 'well if this is so easy to prevent and I don't want to end up losing part of my face, or lose a loved one because we weren't careful about the sun; we weren't concerned about our behavior during the summer and spring or the even the fall and winter. Also, what I hope other people think about is that when the clouds are out; the most harmful rays can penetrate through the clouds and you can get burned in the winter, too, and that's why sometimes you'll see guys going down the slopes and once they hit the bottom they'll put on more sunscreen because the rays from the sun go through the clouds and actually reflect off of the snow, or the water if you're at a swimming pool.

"I once heard from you, Danielle, that down in Australia they have big tubs of sunscreen and that the kids have to put that on before they go out to recess. I was thinking about that a few months ago, when my sister came back from school and she had gotten sunburned from playing outside. It was cloudy and she had gotten sunburned from being outside because she didn't have sunscreen on and [she was burned] around her eyes and nose and on her face. This concerned me [because] the skin on your face is the most delicate. More schools need to have a sunscreen rule: Put it on before you can go out to play. And at home, if we can just have more people put on shirts when they go outside and not just a white T-shirt because that still lets in a lot [of sun]. If we would just remember that being careful about what we wear when we go outside and put sunscreen on, too. In fact, I hear a lot of makeup companies are adding SPF 15 into their makeup and although it's not the best SPF; it's not SPF 30, it's still better than having nothing to protect yourself with. I also tell people my age how sunscreen works; that you have let it soak in and that you have to reapply it. [Sunscreen] really does help and it's a lot better for you than having to deal with the scars on your face when you could have just protected yourself when you were younger. A lot of times they'll say *'but sunscreen gets in my eyes when I get into the pool, or its irritating and I have to wait half hour or 20 minutes before I can go in the water [...]'* I just think, 'you know it's really worth it in the long term and for the rest of your life.'"

On fighting the culture of tan:

"What's funny is that a lot of my friends like to look tan. They like to look like they have been to California or on a cruise or what not, and I actually noticed that its gotten to the point where they will do pretty much anything to think they've got a good tan and stuff like that. I was reading some articles that were on your skincancerribbon.org site, saying what a lot of Americans don't get is that when you get a tan it's actually because your skin has been damaged by the sun. And I just thought that was really interesting because they want to have this tan look, and yet what they really want—what they get is their skin damaged, which can lead to skin cancer. To be tan and get skin cancer it's not worth it. It's not worth to get the scars and to lose part of your face or some of your skin to this when you can prevent it very easily. All you have to do is put on sunscreen; to know what you're doing when you go outside and wear protective clothing, and avoid tanning beds. If you really do want to be tan, there are some really easy things you can do besides going to the tanning bed. You can [use sunless] tanning sprays from the store, and some people say, *'well, I don't want to used them because I'll look orange'*. Well, that's because [they] either [are] applying it wrong or that [they are] using a cheap brand [...] Just don't use a tanning bed. Don't go into the beds because it wrecks your skin. They say you know ours don't have the UVA rays, but they do have the UVB rays, so there are still some risks when you use tanning beds. A lot of times they know about it they know its harmful but I think what they don't know is how it can effect you and a recent survey, I think it was done by the American Academy of Dermatology, or one close to it, that said 38% of teens knew someone that has or has had skin cancer, and its just amazing that they know these people that have had skin cancer, they know the people have gone through it. Yet, they still aren't worried about it. I actually read something where they're trying to pass a law saying if [you are] under the age of 18, you cannot go into the tanning salons. I know a bunch of my friends who go [and they] are 16 and younger [...] but, like I was saying earlier, if you do get tanned by the sun, or by a tanning bed, it's because your skin is damaged. Some people say, *'when I tan my skin looks healthy.'* That's a misconception. It's not true. If you want your skin to look healthy, it will have a healthy glow. You're not going to have it from tanning beds, because it is like being out in the sun, only worse. So, it is a problem and I would like to see something that says minors, at least those under 16-years-old, can't do it. The best would be those 18 and younger, can't use the tanning beds."

On being a "pageant girl":

"A lot of times when you think of pageant girls or pageant teenagers, you think of their bronze skin, how skinny they are, and how they are graceful. [With] the pageants that I'm in, it doesn't matter that you're a size two or what color your skin is; if it's tanned. I have fair skin and a couple of my friends are fair-skinned as well, and they [the judges] aren't really looking at you, just what can you do for the community and what do you have to say. I have noticed that there are a couple of models that aren't bronze. They are pale and they look just fine. And the women in the magazines—they are air-brushed. They are more or less paintings. It's fake. No one looks like that all the time. You don't need to be the model-type to look good. We need to like who we are. We are not all the perfect shade of bronze, or a size two. Everyone has something they want to change."

Kaylan's contributions to the cause:

When Valerie Guild, of the Charlie Guild Melanoma Foundation, and I, were working with Senator Patrice Arent, on a bill asking for mandatory sun safety education for the 2006 Utah Legislative session, Kaylan asked if she could assist us. She approached the entire Utah Senate Education Board and shared the story of her stepfather, Paul, and how skin cancer prevention education she has received from The Cancer Crusaders Organization, coupled with the examples her parents have set about sun safety behavior, has positively impacted her.

> "I think that [mandatory sun safety education] would be a good way to get start getting more schools involved and more people to get that when you are in grade school, since that's one of the biggest times you can get sunburned and that's when easiest time is to prevent skin cancer. I have a couple of friends that are home-schooled, just like I am, and I've told them about this and they are just amazed at how easy it is to get sunburned and how easy it is to prevent it. I think it's pretty easy to teach children sun safety, especially with some of my friends. I have told them about it and they are just amazed how easy it is to prevent it. In my family, what we do is, we all help each other put sunscreen on and my mom, or my aunt, comes and makes sure we have done it correctly, and then we could all go [outside]. It just makes a lot of difference. A lot of the kids will start picking on us about it and they'll start talking about it to their friends. At first they'll just say, *'this is stupid why do we have to do this?'* It does make it a lot easier once they've learned those skills and it is important to put sun safety into them when they're little, because, after a while, they think *'oh, it's easy [to put on sunscreen]! I can do it by myself and not*

have to worry about it.' And when moms are not outside, they learn how to mind themselves and put the sunscreen on [because] it does become a habit. It becomes second nature."

Kaylan's message:

"Teenagers think skin cancer no big deal, but it is a big deal and I would like to see people be more aware of it and just know that there is a danger even if you're going outside on a cloudy day or even in the middle of summer there is still a risk factor, and you still have to be careful when you're going outside and all because of the rays. We need to raise more awareness and see more people being careful about going to the tanning salons, tanning outside by the pool and stuff like that. And mothers, your children need the sunscreen, so just put it on them 20-to-30 minutes before they go outside and play. It helps so much, and it gets them started on good habit. That is all any mother can ask for."

Perspectives on Skin Cancer: Colette Coyne

Interview November 10, 2005

Thank you to the individual who invented the internet (whether it be Al Gore, or otherwise, thank you, nevertheless), and thank you to Alexander Graham Bell for inventing the telephone. If it were not for these modern miracles, I would never have had the opportunity to "meet" Colette Coyne, a mother whose love and devotion for her daughter, Colette Mary Brigid Coyne, whom she lost to melanoma, is evident in all she does.

I first heard of Colette Coyne, the cancer crusader, in May 2005. She was one of three invited speakers at a press conference hosted by American Academy of Dermatology in New York. Among those three speakers included, my friend Natalie Johnson, creator of the National Skin Cancer Awareness Symbol©, a five-time melanoma survivor named Robin Lawrence, and Colette Coyne of the Colette Coyne Melanoma Awareness Campaign. Soon after Natalie's return from New York, I placed a phone call and sent an e-mail to Colette (and Robin). I was in the process of launching an internet radio talk show called "*Conversations with Cancer*", and wanted Colette to be part of my guest line up; to share with listeners the story of her courageous daughter.

Colette's story amazes me. Emotions stir within me whenever I hear Colette repeat the words her daughter told her doctor—*I know my body*—and how she insisted she be thoroughly screened. It was then that she discovered what was ailing her was not a pulled muscle, but rather a deadly disease called melanoma.

On becoming involved:

Colette was the youngest out of our five children, and she was not a sun-worshiper she never used a tanning bed; however she had two blistering sun burns, one when she was about nine-years-old, and we took her to Florida. I put a T-shirt on her when she went in the water. Now, I realize that's not any kind of protection. Colette remembered having another peeling sunburn as a teenager. The doctors said that's all it took to trigger her melanoma. Naturally we don't know what our genetic makeup is, but many people don't have a clue, really, what their pre-disposition is; how susceptible they are to melanoma. Colette had a mole removed, she noticed it was changing. Four years later she would complained about a something hurting her arm, thinking she has pulled something at work [but] it didn't go away. So, she had me take her to the doctor, and the doctor said 'oh don't worry about it. I'm sure it's just a pulled muscle.' Colette, however, said 'no, I know my own body.' She wanted a sonogram.

"Thankfully we had a few months of hope [but] she died two months after that doctor's visit. So, that was the beginning of what I'm doing now. It's because we realized what little we knew about this disease."

On losing her daughter, Colette:

"We started this foundation as a tribute to the courage and love our daughter displayed throughout her life, but particularly toward the end. Although she initially was fearful when she learned of her fate, once she accepted it, she worked to help others to do the same. She insisted we take one last family vacation together [before she passed away]. Although there isn't a day that we don't miss her, we believe her work on Earth must have been completed. Now we work to help others. Colette is guiding our efforts. I get signs of it all the time. I am a woman of faith, and I feel like the Lord will help me. And I really do believe that's what's happened."

On raising a prevention-minded generation:

"Here in Long Island we are trying to promote the EPA SunWise program for education. I think when people start to learn about the dangers of ultraviolet radiation they will begin to think twice about letting their children go outdoors without being protected and they won't permit them to use tanning beds. It is not something that will happen overnight, [but] I think that if we look at the bills we have had passed here in New York—I just really believe that education is really going to make a difference.

"Many years ago one of our sons, he was only about 10-years-old; I was a smoker. I smoked about a pack and-a-half-a-day, and he came home from school one day crying and said 'mommy, please! I don't want you to get cancer!' Well, I didn't stop smoking overnight. Honestly, I hide it from him for awhile, but I thought about how silly it was and stopped smoking. So, if the children get a message [about sun safety and skin cancer] they are going to keep asking their parents about it. How many children say, when they get in the car, say 'mom, dad—don't forget to buckle up now'? Children are great at remembering what they learn and sharing it with others."

On tanning:

"A recent article in the Long Island [New York] newspaper on the outs of indoor tanning quoted some teens and, you know, Danielle, what you have said earlier about young people and their attitude toward melanoma is correct. Many just feel like its not going to happen to them. And that's unfortunate. I don't know how we can combat that mentality, other than on our Web-site we are posting pictures and stories of people who have died from melanoma. This way when somebody is looking at www.ccmac.org they will see its young people this disease is taking. Young mothers and fathers; young 20-year-olds—Perhaps, then will they begin to realize the serious risk they are taking by using indoor tanning beds."

Colette's contributions:

In addition initiating and securing legislation to regulate the use of tanning beds by minors in several counties throughout the State of New York, Colette has traveled extensively giving presentations about the dangers of tanning, as well giving presentations to Parent Teacher Associations (PTA) about counseling parents and caregivers about sun safety for children. Furthermore, Colette is working to implement stipulations that require lifeguards be provided with sun protective clothing and sunscreen, as well as receive sun safety education.

Colette's message:

"I remember that when we were doing [an educational video]. The producer said 'well, we don't want to scare people', and my answer was 'yes we do! This is a scary thing and I think we really need to know about it.' The video has pictures of young people that have passed because of melanoma. Both boys and girls speak on the video. One boy talks about how kids know about cancer, but they think that they it can never happen to them. They think that skin cancer is going to happen to someone else, and yet when it does happen to you it changes your whole life. And hopefully the change in their life is for the better, so that we can help other people so that it doesn't happen to them. Again, it's not going to happen overnight, but if you use the tanning beds it is going to do a lot of damage and you many get skin cancer."

Perspectives on Skin Cancer: Valerie Guild

Interview October 14, 2005

I had the pleasure of meeting this truly incredible woman while attending the first "Play Safe in the Sun" Summit, hosted by the National Council on Skin Cancer Prevention at the National Institutes of Health in Bethesda, Maryland on September 30, 2005. Valerie was a keynote speaker. I was moved by the story of Valerie's daughter, Carolyn "Charlie" Guild, whose life was taken by melanoma when she was just 25-years-old. Charlie, a graduate of Brown University, was preparing to attend medical school when she complained of chest pains. The doctors found no reason or cause for the chest pains Charlie experienced, that is, until six months later when the chest pains returned, and were more severe. A CAT-scan indicated that Charlie had advanced malignant melanoma. She passed away nine months later. Upon hearing Valerie shared this story, my friend, Kathleen, who was sitting to my left, and I looked at each other in utter disbelief. *How does a 25-year-old die from melanoma?* Kathleen and I, both in our 20s, found it painfully arduous to swallow Valerie's words. I passed a note to Kathleen after Valerie's presentation ended and she took her seat among the audience. The note read: "Natalie's brother, Eric, was 21. Valerie's daughter, Charlie, was 25-year-old. How can this be? We need to do something about this right NOW! Cancer Crusaders needs to do more—we need to do more to educate our peers. We have outlived two people who had bright futures ahead of them. When they were beginning their lives, melanoma ended it. Melanoma snatched it all away from them." Since meeting Valerie at the National Institutes of Health in 2005, I have enjoyed the opportunity of partnering up with her on various projects; including two Utah legislative bills advocating skin cancer prevention education and tanning restrictions for minors. Yet, there is still much work to be done.

On becoming involved:

"When this was over, Charlie intended to go out and do something about this disease, but Charlie didn't get that chance. She didn't leave me with much of a choice."

On losing her daughter, Charlie:

"When I went to see her dermatologist for the first time, and when the two of us were alone, I said *'how is this possible? She's 25-years-old?'* I was thinking that he was going to tell me that this was one of those one-in-a-billion-kind-of-things that happened to people. I was floored when he said to me 'well, melanoma is the number one cancer of 20-to-30-year-olds. It is the number one cancer killer of women ages 25-to-29, and Charlie falls right into that category.' Well, I obviously didn't know this and certainly if someone told me that when my children were young that one sunburn—just one can increase your chances of melanoma by nearly 100%, and three sunburns by 500%, I wouldn't have been just warning them. I would have done more to protect them."

On raising a prevention-minded generation:

"I should say that after my oldest daughter Sam was diagnosed, obviously we were all aware of melanoma and all made regular visits to the dermatologists. Unfortunately, Charlie fell into that category of people who have no outward signs of melanoma. So, to me, that even underscores why it's so important why we focus on prevention and awareness. In a case like Charlie's; if we can prevent the disease we won't have to worry how we are going to treat it, and clearly in her case it would have been the only possible way that she could have been saved. I tell people that really there were two moments that made me decide to become involved in this [cause] other than the obvious. The first reason was that after Charlie got her diagnosis, but not her prognosis, she went home and called her friends on the phone. She was 25 but most other friends were older. All of them were very well educated. I could hear her from the other room and, of course, she was teary eyed, but I can tell you I heard her say, 'now, I know its cancer, but don't get upset because nobody dies from skin cancer.' And I quickly realized that if Charlie could believe that, then that is probably what most people believed. I've read the studies from the Center for Disease Control and Prevention which underscore that point, but I didn't need to read the studies, because not only did she believe [that] but all of her friends bought into this and said '*sure, who dies of skin cancer?*' I think about the fact that we obviously teach our children to brush their teeth every morning. We would never expect them to leave [the house] without them getting that done. This is not to say that getting cavities and then, perhaps, loosing your teeth when you are older isn't a serious situation, but why is that we don't take it for granted that after our children are done brushing their teeth that they are going to apply sunscreen to their skin? The reason is that most parents [are] in the exactly same position that I was in [...] we are just unaware of the fact of how deadly this disease is [and] that it really is a young person disease. And it doesn't take someone lying in the sun for years for them to get melanoma."

On tanning:

"There's a misconception that melanoma happens to sunbathers or people who go to tanning salons a lot. That's not to say that it doesn't happen to them, but one burn between ages 0-to-18 is enough to increase your chances of getting it by 100 percent [..] it's not a nice disease."

Valerie's contributions:

Valerie's passion is contagious as she spearheads pivotal, crucial, and vital work on behalf of melanoma research and sun safety education. Among her numerous accomplishments include:

- Indoor tanning legislation under consideration in New York, Connecticut, Washington, California, Maryland, Massachusetts, and Minnesota.

- Legislation mandating K-12 sun safety education, and/or similar education for outdoor workers passed or pending in New York, Texas, California, Florida, Washington, Connecticut, Kentucky, Pennsylvania, Maryland, and Massachusetts.

- Initial work to create a melanoma tissue bank with the participation of the United States Military, University of California at San Francisco, Huntsman Cancer Institute (in Salt Lake City, Utah) and the University of Pittsburgh Cancer Institute.

- Creation of the International Melanoma Working Group, the first international melanoma translational conference, held in Germany in November 2006.

- Initial steps to create a computer-based training seminar geared to pediatricians/pediatric residents in the area of childhood skin cancer prevention.

- Interviews in local and national media including Good Morning America, FOX News, NPR, the *New York Times*, the *Boston Globe*, the *San Francisco Chronicle*, and KCBS-TV.

Valerie's message:

"Last year AIDS research got $6 billion and [melanoma] got $40 million from the government. There really is almost no money out there for melanoma research, and one of the problems is when you don't have research money, you don't tend to attract researchers. I've asked them (the BBYO, an organization Charlie was actively involved with) if they can present this issue in front of all the various chapters, because these are the kids at risk."

Perspectives on Skin Cancer: Robin Lawrence

Interview conducted on August 10, 2005

If I have ever met someone who has been spared or "saved" for a very specific purpose, it would be Robin Lawrence.

A five-time melanoma survivor, Robin exemplifies courage, faith, and grace in all she endeavors, and epitomizes what the band Survivor meant when they penned the anthem *"Eye of the Tiger"*. Robin is the Rocky of the skin cancer community—constantly fighting; a tireless champion for the cause.

Robin's story:

Robin's obsession with the sun and, subsequently with tanning began as a toddler growing up on her parents' farm in southern Indiana. "I seized every opportunity to achieve a deep, dark tan," she says. After graduating high school, she started competing in bodybuilding competitions and began frequenting tanning beds to sport the dark tan look that is very much coveted in the bodybuilding world. Robin's love for tanning grew into a compulsion. Robin only vacationed to sunny destinations, and was rarely indoors, if she could help it. Yet, Robin's sun-worshipping lifestyle soon caught up with her. Robin discovered, in March 2002, that she had melanoma skin cancer. Five years later, she has more than 30 biopsies—five of which were melanoma.

"The question I kept asking myself was 'Why me?' After looking back on my life, I realized I had only myself to blame," Lawrence said. "But I can honestly say that when I was growing up, I knew very little about the dangers of tanning or the threat of skin cancer. It's so ironic that my pursuit of a healthy, active lifestyle was what would eventually come back years later to threaten my life."

Robin on teaching youth:

"I remember you telling me once, Danielle, that nearly 90% of college kids in Utah [you have taught] did not have any prior knowledge of the risk of skin cancer and melanoma. That is exactly what I am finding out in my presentations. I go through everything—I give them my testimonial. I actually show them a video of a young woman who lost her life to melanoma at the age of 24, which they are shocked by when they do watch this [but] then I also go through my own testimonial and then I go through statistics, and then after I go through all of this, students look at me and they're in shock. I tell them, this is the side of melanoma that you don't hear about."

On raising a prevention-minded generation:

"The thing that is concerning me the most is that a lot of the parents are not aware of the dangers of the ultraviolet radiation, so they don't even think about [putting] sunscreen on their children. So, if you can get these kids in the habit of using sunscreen at an early age, that's great because then when they get older they already have that habit with them. And the thing that I hear a lot is, 'oh but it gets in my eyes', or 'it's too wet'. Yet, isn't it better to know you're protecting your skin and you protecting yourself from skin cancer, and, even, that you're helping your skin from aging as much? There was a 50 year study done between 1950 and 2000, and the scary part was the number one cancer percentage increase was melanoma at 1,619%; number two was liver cancer at 295% and number three was lung cancer at 294%. Melanoma continues to be the one cancer that increases in incidence. Melanoma is the number one cancer among women in their 20s [but] it is very preventable. This is why we must educate parents, educate schools—get the message out there that we need to protect ourselves."

Robin on tanning:

"You always hear about the prom specials, the Spring Break specials, and the two-for-one Tuesdays, but this is the dark side of tanning and melanoma that young people really do need to know about it. As of last week, I have had an additional three biopsies. So, that means, I'm now up to 22 biopsies. The scary thing about it is that I have done the damage and now I'm really paying the price. This is going to be the way of my life now. Luckily the biopsies that I had done last week all came back as negative.

None of them where melanoma, but there is always that fear in the back of my mind: *Ok, which one is going to be melanoma? Could this one be or that one be a melanoma?* That's how I got my energy to do what I'm doing. It's my own fear, I thought that I was half-way educated, but I realized how little I knew of skin cancer until I got out there. And as you said before, Danielle, it is a preventable cancer. So, my whole goal is just to tell people about skin cancer and the dangers of tanning, A lot of it is that people, especially young people, don't think its going to happen to them. I really didn't think it was going to happen to me. I remember in high school and looking at these girls with really dark tans. I think the media is doing to that to us, too. They say that's what we have to look like. And, so, I was one of those people who wanted the dark tan, too. That's why I stared to use the baby oil and then, when I started competing in body building competitions, I started using the tanning beds, too. The challenge we have is to just give this information to the people. Let's get people to act on it and let's do something about it. Don't let your children go to tanning beds.

"I'm trying to let these kids know, too, that the sun is more dangerous today then it was 20 or 30 years ago when I was growing up, so because of those dangers of the sun, and the tanning beds, they need to take more precautions. I gave a presentation last week to 700 women, and by looking at the group I could tell that a lot of the women were tanned. I knew by looking at them they used tanning beds and stuff [but] what I did was I polled them. I asked how many of them ever wear a tan and I asked 'how many them had children. At least 90% of these women had children. I, then, asked them 'how many of you let your children ether lay out in the sun or use tanning beds?' And what was shocking was that, the nearly 100% percent of those people let their kids use tanning beds because they have no knowledge that tanning beds are as dangerous as they are. By the end of the presentation; I was supposed to be done by 8:00 PM, but we ended up getting done at 10:30 PM. *I was like what can we do? How can we change this? We need to educate.*

Robin's contributions:

Working as the marketing director for the Evansville Cancer Center in Evansville, Indiana, Lawrence realized that she could illustrate the ugly side of tanning by showing her own personal battle scars from melanoma to help educate others. And that is exactly what Robin has dedicated her life to doing—educating more than 20,000 children and youth about the importance of sun safety, including the dangers of tanning. In her hometown, these presentations are affectionately known as "Pool Patrols".

"When you talk about 'Pool Patrol', it has been a very fun effort. It has been a very enlightening effort. [Pool patrol] is where every week, during the summer, we team up with a radio station and we go and visit different swimming pools [throughout our communities]. When we are at the swimming pool, we talk to [kids] about sun safety and we give them free sunscreen and UV sensitive Frisbees. We, then, demonstrate how to properly use sunscreen. We also demonstrate how ultraviolet radiation works, by using UV sensitive beads. And with these UV sensitive beads and Frisbees that are provided by the Environmental Protection Agency, we teach them that, when these beads turn bright color, that's when they're being exposed to ultraviolet radiation. We teach the kids that what causes skin cancer is UV radiation. The kids know when these beads change colors that is when they need to slap on the sunscreen. So, it's been a fun effort. During the school year, we're into trying to get into the school system and trying to educate children within the school system."

Robin's message:

"The bottom-line for me is that we need to educate. We need to do as much as we can to get the message out about the dangers [of skin cancer] and just try to change our lifestyle [because] not only do we have the dangers of what is happening in our environment, but going to tanning beds is dangerous. Doing that was relatively unheard of 20 years ago, but, for some reason, it's the thing to do. Why do we feel like we have to have a tan? When I was diagnosed, the fear that I had was that I didn't know what my prognosis was. I had a 16-year-old [daughter] at the time and I didn't know if I was going to live long enough to see her finish school. I didn't know if I was going to be here to see her get married or to know her children and that scared me. So, that is what keeps me going. It's a fear that never goes away. The fear is with me all the time. I got melanoma three days before I got my job at Evansville Cancer Center, so I've been able to use my condition personally get more education out to the public. It's sort of a blessing in disguise. I got melanoma [but] I get a chance to educate people."

PART V

Reaching and Teaching Young Adults

- A Case for Service-Learning in Academia

- An Experiment of Application

- Materials and Methodology

- Evaluations and Conclusions

- Results and Testimonials

Reaching and Teaching Young Adults: Effective methods of presenting the message

A Case for Service-Learning in Academia:

Teaching citizenship and leadership development through the application of service-learning, centered on community involvement and personal development, may seem experiential if not idealistic; however, recognizing the varied strengths, abilities, interests, and backgrounds of individuals enables you, as the instructor or manager, to better facilitate learning and growth, and, in turn, develop team unity which thereby increases team productivity in the combined realization of the individual and collective goals and objectives. The idea of incorporating citizenship and service-learning into business management courses and other university curricula, in the effort to breed more competent workers and leaders, is beginning to grow in popularity. Recent pedagogical research studies conducted at several universities throughout the United States reporting measurable success with the application and incorporation of such experiential approaches and theories on leadership development and training.

Perhaps, the pioneer the ideal of experiential learning, particularly with regard to enhancing student performance in (and out) of the classroom is David Kolb who in 1984 authored the best-selling book <u>Experiential Learning: Experience As The Source Of Learning And Development</u> which coined the term "experiential learning theory" (ELT) through the Kolb Learning Styles Inventory model. As a professor of Organizational Development at Case Western Reserve University, where he researches and teaches various courses on learning and development, adult development, experiential learning, learning style, and notably his revolutionary learning focused institutional development in higher education, Kolb is also founder and chairman of Experience Based Learning Systems. Therefore, his interests have given root to the idea of service-learning in the collegiate realm. Based on Kolb's original model on individual learning styles, identifying four distinct types of learning: Concrete Experience; Reflective Observation; Abstract

Conceptualization; Active Experimentation, the concept of implementing service-learning programs on college campuses so as to enrich student comprehension and understanding, and particularly leadership development skills, through citizenship and community involvement was first forged by Campus Compact, a non-profit coalition of more than 1,000 colleges and university presidents working with an estimated 5 million participating students through the United States, with the mission of educating young adults about civic and social responsibility, and leadership development, through service-learning. Yet, what exactly is this term "service-learning" entail? Is it community service? Is it volunteerism? Is it academia? Is it a study in theoretical practices? Service-learning encompasses all of the aforementioned elements.

"Service-learning seeks to engage individuals in activities that combine both community service and academic learning," says Andrew Furco, author of the essay *Is Service-Learning Really Better than Community Service*. "Because service-learning programs are typically rooted in formal courses (core academic, elective, or vocational), the service activities are usually based on particular curricular concepts that are being taught" (Furco 25). According to the American Association for Higher Education (AAHE) service-learning is, as outlined in the National and Community Service Trust Act of 1993, a method under which students learn and develop through thoughtfully organized service that: is conducted in and meets the needs of a community and is coordinated with an institution of higher education, and with the community; helps foster civic responsibility; is integrated into and enhances the academic curriculum of the students enrolled; and includes structured time for students to reflect on the service experience. (Meeropol 2). In sum, service-learning is a standard college credit-bearing program that provides for practical hands-on application of concepts and theories learned through the traditional classroom setting, which, in turn, provides for increased understanding of the material taught through allowing the student to see, first-hand, the relevance of what was taught through "real-life" application. The concept of service-learning is based, to an extent, upon the famous dictum by Chinese philosopher Confucius—*Tell me, and I will forget. Show me, and I may remember. Involve me, and I will understand.*

Truth be told, with service-learning being a relatively new concept being introduced into higher education (hence, the theory of experiential learning and theory), research on service-learning as an effective method of teaching citizenship and leadership development training, on the whole, explicit outline and detail a universally-accepted model or formula for application. Thusly, as Dr. Tamara Ann Waggener, a professor of political science at Sam Houston State

University in Texas, explains, research on service learning often fails to distinguish between service learning projects that increase students' social connections to their communities and service learning projects that deepen students' political connections to their communities. "Certainly the social component of citizenship is important. [The] Universities' commitment to citizenship and service learning may be partially responsible for the high rates of volunteerism seen among today's college students; however, these high rates of volunteerism are not necessarily connected with high rates of political engagement" (Waggener 2). Waggener explains that the lack of evidentiary studies illustrating a direct link to increased community and political involvement, (even increased business acumen in college graduates), and service-learning experiences offered through university programs, proves problematic in making a solid case for universities to adopt policies of requiring service-learning into course syllabi. She refers to a recent article in The Michigan Journal of Service Learning, one of the more comprehensive and well known journals in the area of service learning, which stated "the need to distinguish service learning activities aimed at promoting charity and volunteerism from those concentrating on root causes of social problems, politics, leadership, and the need for structural change" (Kahne 44).

Conversely, a recent study conducted by Dr. Susan R. Madsen, an assistant professor of business management at Utah Valley State College, and Ovilla Wilson-Turnbull, a pedagogical researcher and co-owner of SoftwareFor.org, explain that service-learning applications not only enhances student comprehension of academic topics, but breeds a deeply rooted sense of appreciation and recognition of social issues, structure, trends, current events, and modernity. In other words, the study indicates that requiring students to participate in service-learning, as part of their course major requirements, bridges the gap between heightened awareness and the lack of "pro-action". Madsen and Turnbull published the following results gleaned from their study originally published in the spring 2005 edition of Academic Exchange Quarterly: "Students also wrote, possibly with surprise, that their civic work specifically related to the content of this course, actually helped them learn larger important life lessons. One (of the 25) of the participating students explained.

> 'I work for a successful company and employees get paid pretty well and have fantastic benefits. Yet, these community partner employees made hardly anything. They worked there because they felt good and wanted to make a difference. I found myself wondering, *how can you do that—make a difference in society?* It was humbling. I want to understand this [...]. I think now that I

could really make a difference in this community. I now have the desire [to contribute at work and in the community]'" (Madsen and Turnbull 9).

That being said, Waggener, who, in her essay *Citizenship and Service Learning*, references Madsen and Turnbull's study at Utah Valley State College, and that, combined with additional case studies conducted at Sam Houston State University, concludes that "Service learning has proven to be an important component of the drive towards more civic-oriented students. The vast majority of university initiatives include a strong emphasis on service learning and leadership development" (Waggener 3). She continues, noting that various colleges and universities such as California State University at Monterey Bay require students to complete a certain number of service learning courses before graduation. And other colleges and universities, such as Utah Valley State College, have established centers responsible for facilitating the process of service-learning and leadership development through civic and community involvement through such activities including, but not limited to: acting as a liaison between students and community organizations, maintaining informational resources about service learning, organizing conferences on service learning, and reporting student service learning activity for transcript purposes. (Waggener 3). Among the several dozen students at Sam Houston State University who participated in Waggener's case studies on service-learning, one student's sentiments strike particularly meaningful, if not poignant, in making a correlation between service-learning taught in academia and the application of effective leadership skills. The students volunteered time at the Huntsville [Texas] City Council as part of their service-learning experience:

> "Yes—at first, I felt small in a room of the supposed movers-and-shakers of Huntsville. But with rather concrete data in my hands and with the analysis derived through collaborative discussion with other members of the research team, I felt prepared to deliver a cogent presentation regarding public opinion in Huntsville—and more importantly, I embraced the possibility that this data could shape the future of policy in Huntsville. This was an exercise in authentic learning; I experienced the fruits of my learning not as a result of a professor's assessment of an essay, but rather through the possibility of policy change as a result of my and my colleagues' hard work." (Waggener 5).

Moreover, the aforementioned is sustained by [former] Mayor of Huntsville, Texas, who, commenting on the service-learning performed by participating students at Sam Houston State University, said:

"I'm sure that the project was not only valuable to the City, but also valuable to the students that worked on the project. They got to deal with real issues, present their finding to City Council and City staff, but also see the information they provided resulted in real action on the part of City Council and staff [...] I would like to see these types of service learning projects continue. Both the City and the University have much to gain from this type of partnership" (Waggener 4).

With that, Green continued to say that business leaders, managers, and employers who wish to provide more effective training in the workplace environment ought to consider similar such hands-on training and application as exemplified through service-learning programs in the realm of higher education. After all, leadership, in every sense of the word, is about service. Kathleen Osta, a consultant for the Dallas Human Resource Management Association concurs:

"Leadership is a process of assisting a group to realize its common goals, visions, and dreams. Effective leaders capitalize on the talents and diverse ideas of the group members to formulate and achieve these goals. Leadership involves encouraging a group to develop and grow by creating opportunities for group members to learn from one another through common experiences."

In brief, service-learning marries both traditional textbook learning with practical application, by allowing the student to physically see, in practice, the affect of properly employing concepts taught through standardizes college curricula. As such, students, upon graduating and entering the workforce, are better equipped than their counterparts, to lead and excel in the workplace and are, quite literally, more valuable employees and community citizens.

An Experiment of Application:

Thusly, based on the aforementioned research conducted on service-learning coupled with first-hand involvement with developing service-learning programs for the Center for Service-Learning at my alma mater Utah Valley State College, the idea to devise and implement a one-of-kind skin cancer prevention education program geared towards young adults, came in the form of an experiment in application. The aim: To write original content and develop unique, yet highly effective tools for teaching young adults—particularly college students between the ages of 18-and-30, through the application of a service-learning based approach combined with elements of traditional college courses. If the experiment yielded the kind of measurable results we sought to achieve, and thus proved meaningful, relevant, applicable, effective, and functional, we could then ultimately, as outlined in our initial objectives, present this program to the American Academy of Dermatology for review thereby, upon approval, have this program integrated into the academic curricula of institutions of higher education throughout the United States. The idea: To develop a comprehensive curriculum on both dermatologic and environmental health so as to give college students a strong foundation to thereby teach them about skin cancer and sun safety. The experiment: To create a hands-on, interactive peer education program that trained college students how to teach their peers about skin cancer prevention by combining elements of traditional classroom learning, along with service-learning (community service combined with a credit-based incentive), including, as well, the ease and accessibility of technological resources such as online and video courses.

Materials and Methodology:

The first edition of "ONLY SKIN DEEP?"® Peer Educator's Training and Certification Program included the following materials: A full-color, illustrated workbook that featured 10 lessons divided and categorized into thee separate sections, and accompanied by specifically tailored comprehension quizzes, and interactive activities (e.g., interviewing dermatologists, writing news reports based on surveys conducted among youth on college campuses, hosting sun safety seminars for neighborhood schools, et. al). The first section discussed, in detail, various skin conditions such as eczema, psoriasis, and Actinic Keratoses (AK). Additionally, this section outlined the basic mechanics, structure, and function of the skin, as well as how to properly care for their skin. This included information about how certain chemicals commonly used in popular cosmetics and skin care agents affect the skin. The overall objective outlined in the first section is to provide a clear foundation for the student to better understand how skin cancer develops. After the students learned about basic skin health, we delved into the inherent crux of the curriculum which discussed, at considerable length how skin cancer develops, its correlation with exposure to ultraviolet radiation, and how to properly perform self skin exams to aid and facilitate in early detection. Furthermore, second section of the program on melanoma detection, national melanoma incidence, and treatment options for various stages of melanoma. The third and final section of curriculum focused on ultraviolet radiation and its relationship to skin cancer, effective sun protection (e.g., how to choose a quality sunscreen, and how to properly apply it so as to maximize its efficacy). Additional tools utilized, in juxtaposition with the curriculum, included customized CD-ROMS and Power-Point presentations, shower cards and placards, samples of Blue Lizard Australian Sunscreen, bookmarks and pamphlets published by the American Academy of Dermatology, ultraviolet (UV) sensitive Frisbees from the Environmental Protection Agency, along with pins featuring the National Skin Cancer Awareness Symbol©.

That said, careful review and scrutiny was given to how the "ONLY SKIN DEEP?"® Peer Educator's Training and Certification Program was presented, as a whole, so that the program was made personally applicable, relevant, and meaningful to each student. It was not sufficient to merely disburse skin cancer information to the student, but rather equip them with the tools that facilitated internalization of the information taught and presented through the program. While reviewing methods of delivery, the Kolb Learning Inventory was taken into consideration, along with a critical literature review of the essay *Using 4Mat System to Bring Learning Styles to Schools* (McCarthy 21-27).

The "Kolb Theory", as it is often referred, asserts that a learning style is a student's consistent way of responding to and using stimuli in the context of learning. (Heffler 3).This is ascertained by reviewing the student's response to visual, auditory, and kinesthetic stimuli. While the Kolb Theory is popular, there is little research to validate it. Thusly, a review of aforementioned scholarly piece entitled *Using 4Mat System to Bring Learning Styles to Schools*. In this article, the author identifies fourth individual learning styles, which are illustrated as follows:

- Imaginative Learners: Imaginative learners are oriented toward a concrete experience and reflective observation. These learners have strengths in imaginative ability and posses an awareness of meaning and values. Imaginative learners retain information presented to them most effectively when they are given the opportunity for personal growth, and interpersonal interaction and involvement.

- Analytic Learners: Analytic learners gravitate toward abstract conceptualization and reflective observation. These learners demonstrate strengths in inductive reasoning and creating theoretical models. Analytic learners respond well to information that is based on facts, theories, concepts, and data, and often in traditional educational settings.

- Common Sense Learners: Much akin to analytic learners, common sense learners are oriented toward abstract conceptualization and active experimentation. They possess strengths and talents with problem solving and decision-making. Common sense learners enjoy implementing new information they have learned into immediate, practical use. They want to be involved with hands-on learning that involves experimenting with new knowledge.

- Dynamic Learners: Dynamic learners posses significant talent with developing and executing plans, taking initiative and being willing to engage in new experiences. They are motivated by active experimentation, and value learning how to apply new information; how to transform ideas into appropriate action.

With that in mind, it was mutually agreed upon by all members of The Cancer Crusaders Organization that the first trial run of the "ONLY SKIN DEEP?"® Peer Educator's Training and Certification Program, so as to keep in accordance with our initial objective to offer innovative and effective skin cancer education that is also unique, be presented to our students through a multi-pronged approach that incorporated elements of a traditional classroom setting as well as innovative tools such as internet radio broadcasts, video and television, CD-ROMS and DVDs. As such, the first run of the "ONLY SKIN DEEP?"® Peer Educator's Training and Certification Program began in May 2006 (to correspond with national Skin Cancer Awareness month) and continued, through 50-minute sessions conducted once weekly, until August 2006. Three students participated in the program by "coming to class", three students participated by logging on to live internet radio broadcasts, via a weekly talk show—"*Conversations with Cancer*"—on the Grapevine Talk Radio Network (students simply entered the URL into their internet browser, and clicked on the "Listen Live" icon), and three students participated by listening to audio and visual recordings of the class. Each of the students were required to utilize their workbooks and complete the required assignments as prescribed in their workbooks in order to receive credit for the program; a passing grade of 80% was required to be certified as a peer educator and hence authorized to give skin cancer prevention/sun safety seminars to high school and college campuses (and, in two cases, to earn service-learning credit on their college transcripts). Through this methodology, which included personal testimonies from melanoma survivors, advocates, as well as expert advice given from invited guest dermatologists such Dr. Hayes B. Gladstone from Stanford University, my aim, as the author of the program and course instructor, was to compliment the varied learning styles of each participating student.

Results and Testimonials:

At the conclusion of the experimental run of the "ONLY SKIN DEEP?"® Peer Educator's Training and Certification Program, the students were asked to either complete a final comprehensive exam or write an essay, so as to evaluate their level of learning and comprehension, and to determine if the curriculum was effective. Of the students who successfully completed the course, by which, I mean, completed and passed a comprehensive final exam, an average cumulative of 82% was achieved therefore qualifying them to be, as certified peer educators on skin cancer, as part of The Cancer Crusaders Organization. When each student was asked to evaluate their experience with participating in the program, all comments received were overwhelmingly positive. One of the participants, Hoku, a student at Utah Valley State College, had this to say:

> "I looked forward to coming to class every Friday and hearing what Danielle [the instructor] had to say. Her passion is obvious and her enthusiasm for skin cancer prevention is contagious. I learned so much; more than I thought. I enjoyed the combination of textbook learning, personal interaction and personal anecdotes, along with real-life stories of those who have had skin cancer. I now make sure to check my skin all the time and encourage my parents, especially, my dad to go see the dermatologist. It was a fun, enjoyable experience. I really learned a lot."

Another student, Maile, a student at Southern Utah University, has since worked with the mayor of Cedar City, Utah, (where SUU is located), and the local city council to begin an annual skin cancer awareness month celebration. Maile had this to say about her experience.

> "I spent so much time on this [but] it really helped me. The experience really prepared me. I compete in pageants and my platform is skin cancer prevention education, and participating in this helped me encourage my peers to get more involved. I only wish there were more resources [and] more funding available […]."

Evaluation and Conclusions:

In sum, the idea of a "for the students by the students" approach to teaching skin cancer was well-received. Students responded favorably to having a peer, who was also experienced with teaching skin cancer and sun safety, as an instructor. The combination of traditional college curricula coupled with interactive experiential learning, through an incorporated hands-on service-learning component, provided for an atmosphere that encouraged individual expression while students aimed to meet the prescribed course requirements. Students felt encouraged to speak freely and actively contribute thoughts, ideas, as well as personal experiences, which, in turn, enabled a relationship to form between student and instructor. Students had the opportunity to not only learn from the instructor, but also had the privilege of learning from board certified dermatologists who were occasionally invited to participate by offering expert advice. Additionally, students were given the honor of interacting with melanoma survivors who shared personal insights and reflections, as well as the opportunity to interact with each other and their respective communities. With this multi-pronged approach, students, through the "ONLY SKIN DEEP?® Peer Educator's Training and Certification Program, were given a plethora of avenues to grasp core concepts and principles related to skin cancer that tapped into their preferred methods of learning and comprehension. By catering to the varied learning needs of each student, they were better positioned to personally relate to the information given and apply it in their own lives. Participants in the "ONLY SKIN DEEP?"® Peer Educator's Training and Certification Program were equipped with tools protect themselves from skin cancer and teach their peers, and became anxiously engaged in their communities and emotionally invested in a worthy cause. One participant, Maile, of Southern Utah University had this to say, after passing the course and receiving her peer educator's certification:

> "I have learned more than I could have imagined while writing it. That I assignment I did to make the collages of both tanned and non-tanning celebrities—it was quite interesting who ended up having pictures on both posters. I have since tried to contact the schools [in Cedar City, Utah] to find out about sun safety programs, but with two new schools opening down here, as well as school just starting the principals haven't been very cooperative with getting back to me. So, I am still working on it [...] with schools just starting up again, it would be the perfect time to set up a booth and hand out some sunscreen samples. Thanks for everything you do for skin cancer. I greatly appreciated this experience."

Maile exemplifies what we aimed to achieve through the "ONLY SKIN DEEP?® Peer Educator's Training and Certification Program. Our objective was, with the program, to provide a unique, innovative, interactive, and effective medium by which college-aged students can learn key principles pertaining to skin cancer prevention, but also personally apply those principles by transforming that knowledge into action. Chiefly, our goal at The Cancer Crusaders Organization in reaching and teaching youth, is to educate and inspire; to develop a prevention-minded generation that is proactively involved with teaching skin cancer to others, actively engaged in implementing and supporting necessary measures to reduce of skin cancer incidence and mortality now, and provide the base for the ultimate eradication of the disease in the future. Thusly, it is our intention to integrate this program into the realm of higher education and to have it an accredited college course offered as part of university health and science programs. Whereas numerous sun safety/skin cancer prevention education programs are geared toward elementary and junior high school students, we, at The Cancer Crusaders Organization, recognize an urgent need to teach young adults, as many of them have not been given the opportunity to benefit from such education as children. We must instill within our young adults the necessity of sun protection and dermatologic health so that they, in turn, will instill that within their children and within our communities. Therefore, we seek to partner with the higher education system in satisfying this pertinent, yet previously neglected need to teach skin cancer prevention to our college students—our future parents, employees, and community leaders.

That said, to solidify the utility of the "ONLY SKIN DEEP?"® Peer Educator's Training and Certification Program, the final paper Maile submitted for the course requirements is included in the appendices. Her paper provides a snapshot as to what she gleaned from the course and the possibility of implementation into the university education arena.

PART VI

Author's Personal Anecdotes

- Supporting a loved one touched by cancer
- Coping with the loss of a loved one to cancer

Supporting a loved one touched by cancer

To be completely honest, part of me wonders *who are you, Danielle, to think that you can give good advice about supporting a loved one with cancer?* Admittedly, I am not a licensed social worker or therapist, nor am I an oncologist. I am but merely a 27-year-old girl who started up a non-profit cancer organization. I don't even work full-time in a doctor's office, rather I simply volunteer my nights and weekends teaching people about skin cancer. Moreover, when my mother first told me she had cancer, I sat dumbfounded and paralyzed by silence. Granted, I was 12-years-old and was unprepared to support my mother as she battled with cancer, much less begin to grapple with understanding what cancer was beyond the fact at the mere utterance of the word, my body quaked and shivered. The word "cancer" filled the room with a thick grey, suffocating coldness. In 1993, cancer was not as well-known as it is now, at least not among 12-year-olds. In a paradoxical sequence of events, there is hardly a soul with ears to hear that has not heard of cancer. Much has changed since then, but my experience working with the cancer community throughout the years has not eliminated the feeling of being ill-equipped to write this section.

Nevertheless, I am acquiescing to the incessant pleadings of many friends and colleagues asking me to include personal anecdotes and share my thoughts. Despite that, I am still frantically searching to identify the exact right words to use to express myself. Needless to say, it is a peculiar predicament for someone who rarely finds herself struggling for words. Within me there lies a profound and weighty sense of duty and responsibility to those touched by cancer, which causes me to choose my words carefully. In doing this, perhaps, I can avoid failing people. Therein lies this unquenchable desire to stretch forth my hands and hold their hearts. There is this childlike side of me that thinks if I can hold them long enough and pray for them hard enough that I can somehow eliminate their pain; that I can, through transference, absorb their pain. This surpasses a sense of responsibility; rather it dances within an indescribable, yet tangible sphere that revolves around kinship, loyalty, and devotion. Therefore, I search, still, for the right words to say so that I may speak comfort to their hearts—to your heart.

Hardly a day passes when I don't receive a phone call, an email; hardly a day passes when I am not stopped at the grocery store or approached on the bus ride to work, by an individual who openly shares with me how this elusive foe, known as cancer, has taken an obvious and devastating toll on them. With thoughts racing through my head, there is a silent prayer—*Please, Heavenly Father, take this pain and anguish from them. Fill their hearts with Thy boundless love and heal them. Help me comfort as Thou would comfort.* I, then, cry with them. Alas, the perfect words fail to leave my lips, leaving me to wonder as the hymn says "Have I done any good the world today?" Have I lifted their burden, even for but a minute, and replaced that with a glimmer of eternal hope?

In my attempt to gain insight and thereby be better equipped to support cancer patients and their families, I asked of one of my favorite dermatologists, Dr. Glen M. Bowen, co-director of the Mutli-disciplinary Melanoma Clinic at Huntsman Cancer Institute, to share with me his thoughts. Likely one of the nicest, most sincere men I have ever encountered, Dr. Bowen related the story of losing his dad.

Several weeks later, in reviewing interview tape of Dr. Bowen's touching story, I received an email and phone call from a young woman named Cara who recently lost her mother to melanoma. This, in turn, prompted me to spend a few days soul-searching; examining and analyzing the manner in which I interacted with the cancer community. It is something that I do often, but this time I spent hours on my knees, alone, in my bedroom praying. I gave myself permission to cry, *out loud*, in broad daylight as opposed to muffling my tears in the dead of night when my room-mates were all asleep. My tears drenched my pillows. Emotionally drained, I lay on my bed curled up in a fetal position and playing, in my mind, the thousand faces I have come to memorize over the years. Hours slipped away from me, when suddenly in came my room-mate Melissa, with her luminous smile.

My precious angel-friend, Melissa, walks in to my room and, in her sing-song voice calls out, "Danielle!" "Danielle, what is wrong? Why are you crying?" I remain silent. I was no longer crying at that point, but my red bloodshot eyes and mascara stained pillows were indication enough that I had been crying just minutes prior. I lay still and silent. Melissa proceeds to pirouette across the room and nestle herself at the foot of the bed where she can look at me straight on; like a deer in the headlights there was no way for me to hide my face from her sweet aqua eyes. Melissa whispers, "Tell me everything you are feeling; everything that's in your heart." I told her that I didn't know how; that I was afraid to, but my best friend, with her sweet gentility, intercepts and says "Yes, yes you can. Just let it go, and the words will come." "I am not sure; I do not know how or why I am far better on paper […] I am not used to having someone to pour my heart and soul out to […] For a long time it has been just me and the Big Guy Upstairs". Melissa immediately guessed what I had been thinking about (and subsequently, the reason for the dry, crusty tears plastered across my face). Did I give myself away, or did she simply peer into my soul whereby my heart revealed itself unto her? Did she see the slideshow that is stored there—the slideshow of faces that have occupancy there? Instanteously, the flood gates were, once again, opened. Melissa broke down my walls. "Let me listen. Let me know. Let me in, Danielle," she said.

It mystifies me that as extroverted as I am, that I find it arduous to let people in; I have a propensity to keep my deepest, innermost feelings trapped up inside the confines of soul. My feelings and emotions are sacred, therefore I hold on to them with dear life. Yet, ever since Melissa entered my life my walls have virtually disappeared. They are merely a figment of my imagination. Often Melissa's words ring in my ears: "Don't worry about saying the right thing, just say what's in your heart and let Him take care of the rest." These words are what I refer back to whenever I am presented with a situation where my tongue is crippled and I am without the so-called right words to say to someone touched by cancer. Melissa's words are the ones I reiterate and share; the ones I wish I had said to my mother when she was, faced with cancer, in need of comfort; "Let me in … let Him take care of it and of us." I would have not been afraid to love her, to hold her, to pray with her, nor afraid to be her daughter; her friend.

Coping with the loss of a loved one to cancer

Recently, while out on a run to Panda Express, my friend and fellow cancer crusader, Kathleen, asked me "Danielle, why aren't you a dermatologist. You should go to medical school and become a dermatologist." Amid my laughter, she continued, "You should because you not only know a lot about skin cancer, but you really care about people and you would be so good and so compassionate toward your patients. Why aren't you a dermatologist?"

Quite frankly, this is a question I have been presented with numerous times since starting The Cancer Crusaders Organization. It is perplexing to people when they learn that I do not receive monetary compensation for the work I do with skin cancer and that I develop skin cancer education programs (and write books) in my "spare time, for free." "Why don't you do this for a living, Danielle?" My response: "Because fighting skin cancer, though a passion of mine, doesn't pay the bills. And so I work full-time at my real job and do cancer crusading at nights or on weekends." Truth be told, my current employment situation provides for a healthy balance and makes volunteering my time with the skin cancer community more meaningful, more rewarding, and more personal.

With that said my heart yearns to take people—touched by cancer—in my arms and to crusade along side others who share a passion for skin cancer prevention education. Interestingly, my situation at-present empowers me to do such; it enables me to do pursue endeavors that will improve others' quality of life. It provides for me a necessary sense of balance and sanity.

When someone has lost a loved one to cancer, I am reminded of how precious life truly is and I am filled with a deepened sense of devotion and love for the people in my life. In working with cancer patients and their families, I have discovered that, when I look into their eyes, I get a glimpse into eternity. I am reminded of the twinkle in my best friend's eye and how, when, I look into her eyes, my heart swells with such love and gratitude that it nearly bursts out from my chest. A similar feeling fills my heart when I look into the eyes of someone who has been touched by cancer. I want to take them by the hand and take to the skies; to soar above the Heavens, free and filled with light. It is as though I have been given, however small and miniscule, insight into how Our Maker must feel about us, hence, I become, yet again, a lover of life. In being a lover of life, I love the beauty that exists in it. As devastating it was for me to lose my mother to cancer, and as tortuous it would be if faced with the loss of another person I love; it is this that motivates and inspires me not only to preserve lives by fighting cancer, but to improve the quality of life.

On the other hand, I am not an expert with regard to coping with the loss of a loved one. When my mother passed away, I, regrettably, did not seek the guidance of a professional grief counselor. Consumed by the myriad changes that were occurring around me—from executing my mother's final wishes, to locating my father's whereabouts, to placing phone calls to my mother's friends and associates informing them of her passing, to relocating to another country, it suffices to say that I, at age 15, was ill-equipped and ill-prepared, to face such a series of dramatic changes. While the only noticeable affect in my person performance was that my 4.0 GPA ceased to exist for the remainder of my high school career, the bereavement did, in fact, take a profound toll on me. It would take four years to recognize to what extent, nevertheless it surfaced. And when it surfaced it was as if I had been bludgeoned—nearly to death. Hope Edelman in her book <u>Motherless Daughters</u> explains it well:

"A motherless woman is a walking paradox. At the same time she emits qualities of personal strength, the loss of a mother frequently has damaged her self-esteem, eroded her self-confidence, and evaporated her secure base. This is the fundamental insecurity that makes her scan a room of women and conclude she doesn't fit in. Other women have mothers, she thinks, but I have only myself. Never mind that she has a father or siblings or close friends or a spouse. In a crowd of other women, as a female, she feels alone. Fierce independence and self-sufficiency are her shield, thrust forward as her public display of competence-despite-loss and drawn close as her private protection against the crushing loneliness she otherwise feels. [..] For the motherless daughter, depending on independence isn't nearly as contradictory as it sounds [...] when you lose a mother, there's no longer a fantasy of being able to go home to Mommy. You get thrown head first into the water, and you have to learn how to swim" (Edelman 182).

According to Edelman, who was also orphaned by the loss of her mother to cancer as a child, my reaction to bereavement was not entirely unique or uncommon. "Adults usually start their grief work immediately after a loss, but children tend to mourn in bits and pieces, with bouts of anger and sadness punctuated by long periods of apparent disregard" (Edelman 7). In other words, as a motherless 15-year-old being sandwiched in the midst of a fleeting childhood and an abruptly approaching adulthood, I had to either learn to swim or succumb to the gaping abyss below the surface.

The circumstances that existed after my mother's death, either as an inevitable result of her passing or through choices made by key players associated in one some shape or form, provided little, if any, room to for me swallow the reality of what had occurred, much less digest it or comprehend it. Nevertheless, I wish that, despite my the absence of a built-in support system, that I had the sense, as well as the courage, to, acknowledging and addressing my feelings about losing my mother to cancer, recognize that I needed help and assistance. As it is, I have, eventually, embraced those feelings and learned, at long last, how to live and breathe, and to recognize blessings that have come forth out of the tragedy. In losing, I have gained much, and, in a very real sense, have lost nothing. My mother is with me. She is smiling back at me from the reflection in the mirror. She is with me as I share a laugh with beloved friends, and in every word that leaves my lips. As the days pass and I progressively evolve into an improved version of myself, my mother is there—every step of the way. She has planted the seeds of hope that grow and flourish within my bosom. She has given me life, more than once, and she is in the air that I breathe. My mother remains with me constantly and, therefore, I have only lost an element of tangibility.

In short, when faced with the loss of a loved one to cancer, be not afraid of seeking the assistance of a grief counselor who can properly carry you through the stages of bereavement and thus empower you with the tools to cope. I found myself under a desk one night, crying uncontrollably. After four years of carrying around this monstrous hole in my heart—this void—I broke down. I was then forced to confront the demons loitering around within, and learn to identify myself as a whole, complete person as opposed to this bereaved orphan left incomplete by the loss of her beloved mother. If only I had known how to reach out and recruit the company of friends. If I had recognized that while I may not have felt the need to talk to a grief counselor when my mother passed away, because I was strong, capable, resilient and therefore coping, I, perhaps, could have avoided an exacerbated form of trauma years down the road. Then, again, I was 15-years-old—a child—and hindsight is always 20-20. Fortunately, I have since learned, slowly but surely, to reach out and rally the support of my friends when I need them to sustain me through tragic times of loss and grief. So, to give advice about how to cope with the loss of a loved one, I find myself without a clear, concise definitive answer to give. I am unable to answer that question, because each of us responds to loss in diverse ways; however, I would say this:

Be not afraid. It is okay to ask for help. It is okay to feel. It takes extraordinary strength and faith to realize and admit that you cannot bear it all alone and, as such, seek and obtain assistance. We are human beings, we are vulnerable, and we need each other. Resources are available; there is no need to feel trapped by self-imposed isolation. Our Savior will never abandon us. Life is not a series of haphazard events; rather there is meaning, direction, and purpose to be found.

Therefore, be not afraid. Hope springs eternal. Love extends beyond the veil. And Home is but a breath away.

Afterword

As I moved into my new apartment in the summer of 2006, scared and unsure of who my new roommates would be and how they would affect my way of coming and going, the last thing I expected to change in my life was my skin care. From the moment I met Danielle White that summer, the one thing I did know, however, was that my life would never be the same.

Danielle was entirely independent, confident, passionate, and self-sufficient. She worked a full-time job, ran an award-winning non-profit organization single-handedly, and was in the process of writing a book. Wow! When I learned all of this upon meeting her, I thought: *Perfect! She can be my mentor/personal motivational speaker!* As I got to know Danielle better that summer, I found that she is indeed, a great person to talk to and seek advice from, and a great personal cheerleader. She is also the best friend you could ever ask for. Her example of living is remarkable. When she learns something true, good, and sound, she simply implements it into her life. Learning solid principles motivates her to teach others, so that they, too, can change their lives for the better. I have seen this in all aspects of her life, but most poignantly in the skin care department.

I remember last summer. Danielle wanted so badly to protect us, her friends and room-mates, from skin cancer that she even bought a five gallon jug of Blue Lizard sunscreen for the apartment, complete with a pump dispenser. To the chagrin of interior decorators everywhere, she put it right next to the front door in an effort to make daily application a more convenient part of our lives. Prior to that summer, I had no idea that anyone even sold sunscreen in five gallon bottles! This was just one of the many ways that Danielle showed her immense love for us. That same pure love is at the root of her cancer crusading. During that summer I learned the best ways to stay safe in the sun, as well as some of the best ways to live life.

Thank you, Danielle, for your shining example, for the way you continue to press forward, and for your unending love for this great work and for those around you!

All my best,
Melissa

About the Author

DANIELLE M. WHITE, co-founded The Cancer Crusaders Organization four years ago while a student at Utah Valley State College. Since then, Danielle has been instrumental in developing one-of-a-kind skin cancer prevention education programs aimed at teaching young adults and, in turn, recruiting them to the cause. Danielle is an inducted member of the American Academy of Dermatology's National Coalition for Sun Safety, where she serves on their S.C.R.I.P.T. committee. When Danielle is not volunteering her time with The Cancer Crusaders Organization, dabbling in various entrepreneurial projects and e-commerce ventures, or spending time with friends, she works full-time as a writer and developer for Prosper, Inc. To learn about Danielle's debut book, visit http://onlyskindeepbook.blogspot.com

Appendices

- Dermatologists' Interview Transcripts
- Student Essay
- Bibliography

Dermatologists' Interview Transcripts

<u>Choosing a dermatologist that is right for you</u>
Featuring Dr. Hayes B. Gladstone of Stanford University
(Interviewed conducted by Danielle M. White on March 9, 2006)

DW: What does a dermatologist do; what kind of training do they go through?
HB: Usually if you have a friend or relative. Web-sites, generally, provide good information about how good of a dermatologist a dermatologist is. Staff at a dermatologist's office should be polite and friendly, is a good indication, too. If their staff is short or curt, that's not really a good sign.

DW: What should I look for when choosing? What kind of credentials should they have? Does it matter how many years they have been practicing dermatologic medicine?
HB: Do not go with a dermatologist that isn't a member of the AAD. The AAD makes sure they get continually re-certified and trained. Most dermatologists are board certified. "Dermatologists go to medical school just like any doctor, and after four years of medical school, they do a year of internship, and then three years of dermatologic training to get specialized training in skin diseases, and then take an extremely difficult exam called board certification. In terms of schools, there are many excellent schools, so that's why I say word of mouth referrals. Specialty training usually means they have went through another year of training called a fellowship; American College of MOHS Surgery."

DW: Does it matter if I am a high-risk patient and/or if I am uninsured.
HB: Don't be afraid to open your mouth and ask questions. If the dermatologist doesn't want to answer your questions about insurance, etc., that might be a good indication that that dermatologist might not be the right one for you. Everyone should see a dermatologist. Do your homework, research them.

DW: Does it matter if the dermatologist is published or if they have specific specialties or emphases?
HB: More important to have open-honest communication. May give you piece of mind knowing the dermatologist is well-versed, but it doesn't necessarily mean they are better or worse.

DW: Does it matter if the dermatologist works for a cancer institute, a clinic, or is in a private practice?
HB: No. It matters more their schooling, and if they're licensed, and if they are in good standing with the AAD. "The only exception, I would say, is that if you have a very specific condition such as coetaneous lymphoma, which is a very specific and complex disease, it require different specialties and might be better off going to an academic facility where there are doctors who have extensive training and specialties in those areas."

DW: When preparing for initial visit, what should I do before I schedule the appointment and then ensure first visit gets everything gets started off on the right foot?
HB: "Make sure you have a list of medications. If you have a certain skin condition, that will help the dermatologist determine if it is caused by medications or otherwise. List your priorities; what is important to you. Wear loose fitting clothing. Generally, the dermatologist is going to do a full-body skin exam, and you're going to have to get into a gown anyway. Patients should be prepared for that. If you want to get a good skin check, it's difficult to do that with clothing on. I know some patients are sensitive to that, but knowing it will help the dermatologist get an idea of what your concerns are; any suspicious moles, identification of melanomas, so it is good to be prepared for that and it's good that the dermatologist do that right off the bat. From a doctor's standpoint, part of my job is to provide education. I will always try to provide information about what to look for, the ABCs of Melanoma, how to moisturize and care for your skin, which is very important.

DW: How do I make sense of all the medical jargon?
HB: "Try to educate yourself. I think the internet is pretty good at that. If you have a focused question, you can typically find an internet site that will answer that for you, in laymen terms, and help you with that. Then again, if the dermatologist says something that doesn't make sense, and then stop them right there—say 'I don't understand, please repeat them in language I can understand.' Just smile. They will usually laugh and realize they were talking over your head and re-explain things. If the dermatologist has left the room, there's usually a nurse. Ask the nurse. You can also get their email address, and send them a request for further explanation. Sometimes writing things down helps the dermatologist explain things in different ways that are easier [for the patient] to understand. If you repeat your question, the dermatologist will usually be very

understanding [if they are made aware] that they haven't been answering your question well, and will find other ways of clarifying everything. The average time a dermatologist takes in explaining things is only 23 seconds, so interrupt, repeat questions, talk with the nurse, or send an email. I think that's where email comes in handy. Often time the patients don't want to come across as annoying, or take up too much of their dermatologist's time, but it helps the dermatologist realize that they need to do more to help the patient understand."

DW: How can I maximize my follow-up visits? How can I get my family members and friends into the dermatologist?
HB: "First of all, you should have a yearly skin check, unless you have other skin issues, such as psoriasis, or if you have had skin cancer, you should go in every six months. I always tell my patients o become friends with my staff, particularly the person in charge of my scheduling, and tell them you really need to go it. There are key words to say: 'I have a spot a changing greatly.' Since that is usually a key sign of melanoma. You'll probably get in sooner than later, if you use buzz words."

DW: It has been my experience in being apart of The Cancer Crusaders Organization that men are especially difficult to convince. I have women call me or email me almost on a daily basis asking me what should to do encourage their husbands and fathers to see the dermatologist; what I, as a female skin cancer activist, do to encourage men. As a man, and more specifically as a male dermatologist, can you shed any light on why most men are reluctant to visit the dermatologist?
HB: "Guys are hard to recruit. Many guys haven't gone in to see the doctors in years. Yet, men are very visual. Show them pictures of skin cancer. Have them surf the net. It drives the message home, seeing pictures of scars and skin cancers. AT this point, skin cancer, unfortunately, affects 1 in 5 Americans, so the odds are of knowing someone with skin cancer is really high. Men will want to go to the dermatologist as long as they know the skin exams won't hurt. Start early. Educate people when they're younger and they will have a better chance of going in as an adult."

DW: When should I start going to the dermatologist for skin exams?
HB: "Generally, things start to change at puberty. There are more skin conditions being seen in children, such as dermatitis. But, generally, once hit puberty; go in because that's when moles start changing. Parents can take their teenagers

in and get an idea of what is normal for their skin, and what's not, early on. Many teenagers tend to go into the dermatologist anyway for acne. Because of the prevalence of skin cancer, I'm seeing skin cancer more and more in people in theirs 20s. Later in life you will be glad you went to the dermatologist every year when in your 20s, because your skin will look a lot better in your 50s."

DW: Are there any additional pieces of information or points you would like to address before we go off the air? Are there any key points that I might not have addressed during our discussion today?

HB: "The point I would want to emphasis is that choosing a dermatologist is not easy. When it comes down to it, [is it is imperative that you] form a relationship with them—one that you want to have for life; a lifelong relationship. I always try to find out about their lives, if they have children, what they do, what books they have read, and establish a bond. If you don't feel that, don't feel like you're going to offend the dermatologist if you seek another one because it is important that you feel that you have got a sense of satisfaction. After two visits, if you haven't got a good feeling from that dermatologist, then seek another one—ask your friend for referrals, too. Any relationship enriches your life."

Facilitating effective two-way communication between dermatologist and patient
Featuring Dr. Glen M. Bowen of Huntsman Cancer Institute
(Interview conducted by Danielle M. White on March 9, 2006)

DW: Skin cancer is so preventable, but so common, It doesn't need to be common. Yet, because it is preventable, I feel there's an element of hope here and that we can actually do something to conquer this disease. First of all, I would like to you about; I have a lot of college students—I work with college students quite often—and they say, "Well, how do I really understand my melanoma risk? Is everyone at risk? Is it largely hereditary? Is it mostly environmental?" As a dermatologist, what would you suggest I tell them?

GB: "Well, the first thing to say is that melanoma is the deadliest skin cancer, but it actually is a minority of the skin cancers. The more common skin cancers combined account for over half of all cancers diagnosed in the United States, so over 50% of all cancer in the United States is skin cancer, and the vast majority of those are from the sun, and therefore are preventable. Melanoma can occur in places that are not sun-exposed, like the soles of the feet, inside the mouth, on the scalp, in hair-bearing areas—but most of them are going to occur directly because of sun exposure."

DW: Back tracking slightly, will you briefly describe to our listeners what skin cancer is and how it is identified and what to look for—signs and symptoms?
GB: "The vast majority of skin cancer, from the patient's perspective, are going to be sores that don't heal. Some of them might be sores that heal short-term but then they break down again, and in my young patients they're often perceived as a pimple. They have a spot, it doesn't seem to get better, it finally heals, but then it breaks down again. So, the vast majority of skin cancers are basically going to be a sore that persists and doesn't quite heal. Melanoma is usually going to be identified as a mole, usually brown or black. Rarely, they can be red. And so, pretty much, for melanoma, if the patient keeps in mind that if they have a mole that does not look like their other moles that most definitely needs to be evaluated by a dermatologist."

DW: How do melanomas start? How does a sore become a melanoma, and why is it so deadly?
GB: "Well, melanomas—about 70% of them are de novo, which is a medical term which means that they start spontaneously as a new mole. About 30% will be a mole that you have that changes color or shape. The reason melanoma is deadly probably is because embryologically, they're derived from the neural cells. The first thing that forms when a fetus is forming is what's called the neural tube, and those cells are fantastically capable of migrating to other parts of the body, so when a melanoma forms it doesn't have so many steps backward to go until it behaves like an embryonic cell and can travel to the lungs, the liver, the brain and set up shop, and cause growths there that can lead to death.

"The other skin cancers, which are more common, are more late-term tissues, in other words, they're developed much later during embryology, and so they're not as aggressive. They have to back up a lot more steps before they become extremely migratory. So most of those are very easily treatable with surgical excision, the problem being a lot of them occur on the face, so to remove them—it's quite disfiguring, especially if they're on the nose or the ears"

DW: Yes, that is an excellent point, Dr. Bowen. I've worked with [people] in the skin cancer community where they've had facial disfiguration because of their melanoma surgery, and it's been actually quite traumatic for them.

GB: "Yeah, if they're caught early, the surgeries are not terribly disfiguring, but a lot of the skin cancers grow a little bit like the oak tree, and they'll send down a root structure that's invisible on the surface of the skin, so when we go in and remove them microscopically, the defects can be very profoundly large compared to what it looked like on the surface. So early diagnosis, of course, is the key."

DW: Definitely. I can't emphasize that enough. Early detection is the key. So, what could we tell those listening about melanoma so our communities can better reduce their chances of ever having to be diagnosed with it, or at least know what to do to catch it early?
GB: "Well, melanoma is kind of an interesting skin cancer, relative to the other types, because it tends to occur in areas that are usually sun protected, for example, the back, the abdomen, and in women, the calves. So we don't know for sure, but we think one reason might be that these are spring break cancers. In other words, you have parts of your skin that are protected during the winter, and then when you go to Cancun with your college room-mates and get peeling sunburn. We also that melanoma, in particular, is a lesion of childhood sunburns. So the main thing to say for young people and for parents of young people is to—beg, borrow, or steal—avoid sunburn."

DW: Well said. I would add to what you just said, Dr. Bowen, that we must remember and remind others to properly use sunscreen, wear sun-protective clothing. This is especially important for children since 80% of one's lifetime sun damage occurs before age 18.
GB: "The majority of the [sun] damage that leads to melanoma probably happens before we graduated from high school. And why that is might be a combination of the fact that most of the recreational sun is acquired when you're a child, it may be that the skin of children is less able to protect itself from the harmful effects of ionizing radiation, but the bottom line is that it is critical that in the years before one graduates from high school, that seems to have the greatest impact on your future risk of getting melanoma."

DW: What about high-risk melanoma patient? I have some friends who are considered high-risk melanoma patients. What does that really mean, other than the obvious?
GB: "Well, the things that we definitely know confirm much higher risk of melanoma are having it in your family. So if you have a first-degree relative—for example, your parents or a sibling—that have had melanoma, then we think it on

average increases your risk by a factor of two, possibly three. So that's number one; number two is the number of moles that you have. So it doesn't mean that the moles that you have are going to turn into melanoma, but the people that make lots of moles statistically are more likely to make a melanoma. The third thing is, just flat-out, the number of peeling sunburns you've had; just the raw number of sunburns is very statistically significant. And then, your skin type; red hair, blue eyes; blonde hair, blue eyes confers a much, much higher risk than brown eyes, olive skin."

DW: Everyone, however, is at risk for melanoma, regardless of their skin type or family history. Is that correct?
GB: "Yeah, that's right. In fact, Bob Marley, the Jamaican reggae singer, died of melanoma that occurred on his foot, and it metastasized to his brain. African-Americans, Navajo, Asians, Hispanics, they all can get melanoma, but of course they get them at a lower incidence than a Caucasian would."

DW: I'm glad you said that, Dr. Bowen, because my friend Ani, who is Navajo, laughs whenever I tell her to put on her sunscreen. She says, "I am brown, Danielle, I'm not going to get skin cancer," and now I'm going to have her listen to this and say, "Dr. Bowen said that is not true."
GB: "No [that is not true]. I've treated melanoma and other skin cancers in people with very dark skin"

DW: So, I'm concerned about melanoma, and I want to protect myself and my loved ones. I've found a dermatologist, [but] what can I do to make sure that I'm on top of it, so to speak? In other words, what questions should I be formulating in my head in preparing to visit the dermatologist, and how do I to be following up [with my dermatologist]? What would suggest that I do to be my best advocate and thus prevent myself from ever having to deal with melanoma?
GB: "Well, that's a great question, and the answer is a self skin exam. The problem with melanoma, to a large extent, is that most of them are going to occur on the back, and are not very easily recognizable by the patient. So, it really pays high dividends to examine your skin once a month. I always tell my patients, 'Just for consistency, pick the first day of each month, and when you get out of the shower, get a hand-held mirror and look at your back using the bathroom mirror for the double reflection.' If you do that, it's pretty easy to see your back, and most melanomas. I should really emphasize [melanomas] are not difficult to spot, you know; they really look different from the other moles on the body. The

problem is, especially men, they just tend not to pay attention. So, they come in and then, you know, they're caught completely by surprise when the doctor finds something on the back that otherwise went unnoticed. So, the self skin exam is extremely important, and I like it when my patients actually make a laundry list. They'll look at their skin and say, 'This is a little bit unusual,' and when they come in, they make sure that I go through the check list and answer their questions as to what the lesion is. Most of the time, by the time you get to the third time that you've seen the patient they're pretty comfortable with what the different lesions are on the skin. Because there are lesions that are extremely common, and it helps to educate the patient as to what those are so that they know not to worry about them."

DW: That is an excellent idea. So, speaking of suspicious moles, Dr. Bowen, if you find a suspicious mole on one of your patients, how do you prepare a patient for that? Naturally, you will want to excise it and make sure it's gone [but] how do you prepare them for that procedure—what's involved? What happens after it has been excised?

GB: "Well, if I think it's a melanoma, I try to tell the patient as gently as I can that I have a high suspicion that it's melanoma. The word is a very loaded word, and people actually tend to freeze, like a deer frozen in the headlights of an oncoming truck. So, since I know that, I try to explain to them that. So, I tell them that I'm going to remove it today and find out if it is or it isn't, and once I know that, then I'll do the proper surgery to remove it, because we don't know how much skin to take or whether or not to sample lymph nodes until we know how deep the melanoma is. The biopsy is very simple; there's very little pain involved. We inject it with litocane, similar to what the dentist might use for a dental procedure, and we biopsy it and either stitch it up, or sometimes we just leave them open and put a bandage on, and they're not terribly painful. Once we have the pathology report, they will give us a measurement of the melanoma in depth, which is measured in millimeters. So if they're very thin, we do a re-excision, and sew it up. If it's deeper, then we might sample lymph nodes to make sure that they're not involved with the cancer, and do a little bit wider and deeper excision."

DW: Are there different kinds of excisions or different kinds of biopsies, and is there one particular one for different stages. Does stage matter?

GB: "There is an assortment of biopsies, but they're not terribly important. The main thing is, we try to remove most or the entire tumor, so that the pathologist gets a good look that's going to be representative of the whole tumor. And they're not very morbid. They're quick; they take about five minutes in most cases, and the patient's in and out. A lot of patients won't go because they're simply afraid of having the biopsy, and they're more afraid of what the biopsy might tell them. The irony is, the fear of having a minor surgery can keep them from having a life-saving treatment."

DW: That is true.
GB: "Yeah, it seems obvious, but you'd be surprised at highly intelligent people that will postpone a very trivial thing to the point of where they have a life-threatening disease just because they just didn't want to be inconvenienced."

DW: There is that element of fear, but on the same token, it's so much better to know. I personally feel that knowing brings peace of mind, and so it's worth it. Would you agree?
GB: "It's a pretty common human experience that there's a lot of things in our life that we dread doing, and that creates a great deal of anxiety [but] once we do it, we ask ourselves, 'What was I worried about? It wasn't that bad.' And that's recapitulated through every aspect of your life. In this case, it actually could *be* your life. So, it is important to not postpone having something looked at if it's unusual."

DW: And if a patient is anxious and concerned; they kind of feel they can't do it because they are afraid—is there anything that their friends or their loved ones can do or say to help them overcome that and go through with the procedure?
GB: "Oh, definitely! I'll give you an example. I had a man in this week with a melanoma on his scalp. He'd had it for a year, and his wife had been trying to get him in to the doctor for a full twelve months before he finally consented to come in. And then, you know, the biopsy took five minutes, and then when he left he said, 'That was a lot easier than I thought it would be.' Often, women, for whatever reason, as a group tend to be much more likely to come in, but men are very difficult to get to come in, and so it's usually they're going to come in with a loved one with a gun to their head, so to speak."

DW: That does often prove to be true.
GB: "It's one of those things where tough love is needed. You know, if there's something on a loved one that's really important, you know, sometimes it takes a little bit of muscle to get them to go in and get that appointment."

DW: I have to chuckle at that because that is so true. I have seen that time and again. Even talking with my college students, the girls are more apt to say, 'Okay, Danielle, I did my self-exam!' They get excited about it, whereas the guys remain silent and reluctant. I don't know why that is, Dr. Bowen. I still haven't figured that one out yet.

GB: "Well, I haven't either. One statistic that's very interesting is that 50% of melanomas in men are initially found by a woman. So, half of the melanomas that occur in men are found by women. In women, 4% of their melanomas are found by men. So, that tells you lots of things [and] one of them is, men are looking [but] they aren't looking at the right stuff, if you know what I mean."

DW: True, so true. So, revisiting the issue of biopsies. What happens? You have said that it (the mole) gets tested, and it goes to the pathologist. Yet, I have heard—fortunately, it hasn't happened to anyone that I'm close to, but I've heard of this happening—occasionally the lesion that has been removed either gets lost or misplaced or thrown away, and then they (the patient) never hears about it again. How can a patient make sure that the dermatologist, and the pathologist, is going through procedure and that they will get the information back on their biopsy?

GB: "Well, you have to take some responsibility as a patient. Me being a doctor, I've also been a patient, and I can't stress enough that you have to take some responsibility. This isn't going to [an amusement part] and getting in the roller coaster and having the seatbelt clashed and you just go along for the ride. You have to take some responsibility for what's going on. It is very rare for a lab specimen to be lost or mislabeled, but there are cases where patients didn't receive the letter, or they moved, or somehow we weren't able to contact them with the biopsy results and we literally can't find them. And so, you know, it is some responsibility of the patient to make sure they know what the pathology result was. We have had several legal cases that I've been asked to consult on, where the physician removed the lesion and did not submit it to pathology. In other words, they were so confident that it was a benign lesion that they threw it away. So, as a patient, you have every right to insist that when something is removed from your skin, that that be submitted to a pathologist. And I would encourage the patient to be so bold as to ask the doctor that. My patients ask me that a lot more than you would guess; they'll say, 'Well, you are going to send that to the lab, aren't you? You aren't going to throw that away?' And I always reassure them and show them the specimen in the bottle, that 'Yes, this is going to go to a pathologist for evaluation.'"

DW: And that's good for your patients, too. I don't think that we, as patients, realize or remember that we do have to take some responsibility. We can't lay everything on the doctor's feet. Our doctor is going to take care of us, of course; a dermatologist is going to do everything that he or she can to protect us, but at the same time, you've got to open your mouth and ask those questions, and not be afraid to. And if your dermatologist is a good dermatologist and you have a relationship with him or her, they are going to allow you to ask questions like that. So, that's an excellent point I'm glad that you brought up, Dr. Bowen.
GB: "I would say, if they don't allow questions, or if they seem to be offended by questions, you need a different doctor. Because that's just not acceptable."

DW: That's right. If you can't ask questions, you need a new dermatologist, right away. Okay; so the excised mole goes to a pathologist. Heaven forbid, it comes back, and it is a melanoma. How is that relayed back to the patient? How does the dermatologist reassure the paint and to help them grapple with that?
GB: "Well, there's no good answer, Danielle. That's a phone call that I hate to make, because it's very reproducible. You tell the patient (I call them), and there's a sort of a silence, and then a sort of an 'oh no.' And you know that they're seeing—their whole life flashes before their eyes, and they're thinking about their children, and what's going to happen to the kids; who's going to take care of them.

"Probably the biggest mistake that happens at that point is after I say, 'you know, we're going to remove it, you have a very high chance of having a complete cure with surgery,' they immediately log on to the internet. And the greatest mistake that happens is that they confuse the stage of the disease with the Clark level. All that means is that there is a roman numeral given with the diagnosis that is sort of an anatomical measurement of how deep the melanoma is in the skin. And if they hear about the Clark level; a lot of patients get their hands on the path reports, so they look up on the internet and they go by stage. The stages of melanoma are one, two, three and four, one being in the skin and thin, and four being in distant organs, you know, with about a 10% five-year survival. I can't tell you how many patients have come into my clinic absolutely emotionally distraught, as is their family, because they think they have stage four disease. They think they have a 10% chance of being alive in five years, when in fact they have a 95% chance of being alive in five years.

"The internet is not policed by anybody; there's good information and there's terrible information, but most of the time with the initial diagnosis, the patient doesn't have enough information to read what is on the internet and draw proper conclusions. There is a time for the internet, but it's not right when you get your diagnosis. So, I encourage patients to trust their dermatologist to give them accurate information, wait for that interview when you come in for the post-biopsy discussion, and after that, the dermatologist can direct you to Web-sites that are legitimate, and tell you what information is relevant."

DW: That is very good, and very helpful, to know, Dr. Bowen. It is true. Trust your dermatologist. If you have that in place to begin with; if your dermatologist tells you that you have melanoma, because you already trust him or her, you will continue to trust them. The time to trust your dermatologist would most definitely be in a situation like that, when you are diagnosed with melanoma. That said, do dermatologists ever counsel patients on how to break the news to their family, and how to seek support—emotionally and physically—once that diagnosis has been made?

GB: "Once we have the diagnosis, when they come to Huntsman Cancer Institute, I make an assessment in the room, basically of the patient's emotional status and the family or the people that come with the patient. It's really important when possible to bring family or friends because the patient, quite honestly, is not going to remember much of anything that I tell them. They're just not. It's human nature; they're frightened, they're intimidated, and they're usually thinking about 10 steps ahead of what I'm saying. If a family member is present and can hear the discussion, they often can talk to the patient down after the interview.

"The second thing is, we have professional counselors at Huntsman Cancer Institute and so we try to get patients hooked up here. And that's very helpful for the counselors to talk to the patient and say, 'look, here are some very reproducible human emotions that you're likely to experience: anger, resentment, fear and people go through fairly reproducible stages.'

"I kind of view a cancer patient similar to those poor guys that went to Vietnam. I think one of the great stressors for the vets that I've talked to is they didn't know who the enemy was. A little man might be carrying some rice on his back coming down the street and could drop a grenade in their backpack and blow them up to pieces. They didn't know who the Viet Cong was and who wasn't. With cancer, and not just with melanoma, but with cancer, in general, it's kind of a fear of that unknown that's overwhelming for patients.

"So, what we (the dermatologist and the counselor) try to do mentally is say 'You can't eat an elephant in one sitting. Nor do I want you to attempt to do so. So, that is when my job as your doctor is to carve the elephant up into small steaks and we'll give them to you one at a time. So, here are the short-term goals and here are the long-term goals.' I try to paint the picture of what the immediate task is and what the long-term task is for them. And once I have done that, it's a little bit of Zen philosophy that you, as the patient, just have to concentrate on putting one foot in front of the other and concentrate on the first task at-hand. Most patients, if they can just concentrate on the thing right in front of them and give it their full attention, they do better emotionally than people who try to swallow the whole thing whole at the first visit."

DW: This is excellent information. I appreciate what you said, Dr. Bowen. With regard having a family member or friend in the room at the same time—how can they member help that patient throughout the entire process, from initial diagnosis to treatment and survivorship?
GB: "Well, I think this would be a little bit of restating the obvious, but I think that the family members have to be very careful to do their best to understand what it's like to be in the patient's shoes. Sometimes family members come in and they're so focused on how the cancer's going to impact them that the patient starts to become irrelevant. It's all about me, you know what I mean? So it's important to not jump in and butt in and sort of take the spotlight onto yourself, which is shockingly common. And I don't think it's that people are selfish, or that they're conceited, it's just that they're frightened. And at that point I think it's important to remember "okay, this is the patient. This is the person I have to support. What kind of questions can I ask that are likely to be helpful?""

DW: And that is a good point. I wouldn't have thought of that happening, but I guess that would make sense, especially if it were maybe a spouse. If I was married, I would be thinking *oh my goodness, what am I going to do without my husband, the father of my children?*
GB: "Yes, and it puts added stress on the patient if the spouse is falling apart like a house of cards. And if it happens, it happens; that's okay, we have a counselor to help couples sort through that, but it's a time when strength is needed and when support is needed. It's like the verse in Ecclesiastes: there's a time for everything, and a season for everything. That's the time to step up to the plate and be a support."

DW: And what you are close friends with someone who has been diagnosed with melanoma, and they don't really want to talk about it, but you're concerned? You love them and you want to be there for them, but they don't want to talk about it. How can we be supportive of them without forcing them to talk about it; to be supportive without being obnoxious or interfering?

GB: "Oh, absolutely. When my father died, I'd not lost a person in my immediate family, and I had no idea how I was going to react until I was going through it. Nor did I have any idea how my siblings were going to react. It was quite shocking to me, the different ways that the five of us handled my dad's death. We all needed different things, and I think that that takes a great deal of empathy to try to know a person well enough to try to see what they need, and not force-feed. You know, like say 'Oh, I don't think you're facing up to this, you need to really talk this through.' Well, they may not really want to; they may not be ready to, but what might be helpful is saying, 'Gosh, you know, you might need some time to sort things out, or you might need some time for appointments. Can I set up babysitting for your kids?' 'Can I mow your lawn?' 'I know you've got a lot of stuff on your plate. Is there something I can do to help out?' There's a quote by Jon Huntsman Jr. in our Cancer Institute that basically says, the real value of being a person close to a person with cancer is to help ease their burden. So whatever it takes, you just kind of need to know somebody and ask yourself a series of questions of *what is the best way, for this person that I can help ease their burden.* And often it's the day-to-day things; it's the picking the kids up from school, it's the groceries, it's the logistics of getting to a doctor's appointment and who's taking care of things at home. So I don't have any good answers, Danielle, but those are just some broad suggestions of keeping in mind trying to ease somebody's burden."

DW: That was an excellent answer, Dr. Bowen, thank you. When my mother was diagnosed with cancer, I was just 15-years-old. And she was a single parent, I was her only child, and when her friends would do things like that—because my mom was extremely introverted; she wouldn't really talk about how she felt or what her treatment was like or anything like that—but she had these friends who wanted to help her; so they would say to her "Cindy, we want to do things with you," and that helped, just you said, Dr. Bowen, but those who said, 'Cindy, you're not talking about this, you're in denial' would cause her to retreat inward. I thought that was an excellent answer, personally, Dr. Bowen. So, thank you.

GB: "Well, everybody's different, and unfortunately there isn't one approach that's going to work for each person. Sometimes you don't say the right thing and you come across as being insensitive, but that's better than not trying anything at all. And I think there's some responsibility for the patient; it's an extremely difficult time, and we need to cut them slack for moments of emotional outburst and probably getting angry easily, but I think it is important that if you are a patient that has cancer, to try to understand the awkwardness of loved ones that want to help but don't quite know how to help. I think that it's really helpful if you'll *ask* for help, and say, 'gosh, you know, it would really help me out if you did blank,' and most people will be so grateful to you for having articulated something, that they will just be eternally grateful."

DW: That's very true. Dr. Bowen, I appreciate everything that you do and how well you state things, and most importantly the compassion that you have for people. It's very obvious when I see you speak and very obvious here on the show, too. I appreciate that. I wish there were more dermatologists that were not just scientifically savvy, but had that compassion too; that they could connect with people. So, thank you, for sharing your knowledge.

GB: "Thanks, Danielle, for taking an interest. I'm extremely grateful, as are the other physicians over at the Institute, for the time and effort you put in getting the word out. It's one of those cancers we can do something about and we just don't have to have as many people dying as there are."

Understanding your role in reducing your risk for skin cancer
Featuring Dr. Clay J. Cockerell of the American Academy of Dermatology
(Interview conducted by Danielle M. White on August 26, 2005)

DW. What is skin, what is it made up of, and how does it work? What is the primary function and purpose of the skin?
CC: "Basically your skin is your protective barrier from the outside world. It's kind of like a how a turtle has a shell, so our body has skin. It protects us from many different things, particularly the elements. Basically, your skins function is to protect you."

DW: What is skin cancer?
CC. "In sum, skin cancer is the uncontrolled growth of immature cells in the skin. Skin cancer is a situation where the cells in the skin have been damaged, and, unfortunately, just like any cell in your body that has sustained damage can lead to cancer. And cancer cells grow very rapidly thus cause a potentially life threatening situation in some cases. So, in the case melanoma, a very serious and

potentially deadly form of skin cancer, it is a situation where the pigment produc-ing cells in your skin [melanocytes] have sustained prolonged damage."

DW: On our very first show we talked about the three different types of skin can-cer—basal cell carcinoma, squalors cell carcinoma, and melanoma. What are the key signs and symptoms I should be looking for each of this specific types of skin cancer? How are they similar and how are they different?

CC: "Basically, it is as the story goes: If you have a bump on your skin that comes up or a lesion on your skin that is bleeding, go to the dermatologist immedi-ately."

Understanding your risk for melanoma; advances in melanoma research
Featuring Dr. Sancy A. Leachman of Huntsman Cancer Institute
(Interview conducted by Danielle M. White on September 5, 2005)

DW: The first question I actually have for you is: unlike most cancers such as breast cancer, skin cancer is typically said to be caused by external environmental factors, such as overexposure to UV rays. Yet, there must be, to an extent, a level of hereditary involvement with one's likeliness of getting melanoma. Would you be willing to tell us about that relationship—the familial relationship versus the environment, and talk a little bit about that p16 gene I keep hearing so much about.

SL: "Sure. Well, it's a pretty complex interaction between the genes and the envi-ronment in skin cancer, and I think it's really important first that we make it really clear that there's a major division in types of skin cancer. There's mela-noma, which you've been speaking about today, and then there's a non-mela-noma skin cancer. The link between ultraviolet light, sun exposure, and non-melanoma skin cancer is really pretty clear. I don't think you'd get any disagree-ment from anyone about the role of burning and ultraviolet light in the develop-ment of non-melanoma skin cancer.

"I'm just going to deal with the genetics of that real briefly, because it's impor-tant there, too. Even though the non-melanoma skin cancers are very definitely caused by sunlight, there's also a component of genetics that puts people at more or less risk. I think everybody knows of a typical red-headed, freckled-faced, very fair-skinned person who always burns and never tans; those kinds of people, their exposure to ultraviolet light causes much more damage for some reason in their skin than a person who is very olive-complexioned, or has a very Latin back-ground, or a black patient. Those people, the same amount of ultraviolet light does not do the same amount of damage to their skin as it does to that fair-skinned, freckle-faced person. So even though, yes, it is the sun exposure that's causing the problem, it's also because of the genetics that made them who they are that those with fair complexions who are more vulnerable to the sun. So there's a dynamic interaction between the genes and the environment there.

"Now, in melanoma it's a little bit different, so we're I think going to spend more of our time today talking about melanoma. Melanoma probably has a larger component of genetics in it to some extent than environment. We do believe that the ultraviolet light does predispose to melanoma, but the data on that is much less clear, and we're not certain what form of ultraviolet light it is. Some investigators believe it's the same wavelength, the UVB rays that cause most of the damage in non-melanoma. But there are some investigators that think that's not true, that it's the ultraviolet light A, or that it's not necessarily the daily exposure, but it's really the exposures where you get the bad burns that are the ones that cause melanoma. I guess the bottom line is that there's still quite a bit of controversy surrounding how and why ultraviolet light causes an increased risk for melanoma. We do know, though, that those people who have a strong family history of melanoma, so somebody who has three or more members in the family who have had melanoma in particular, those people are at the highest risk of developing melanoma of all the people in the world. So there is something that's running in those types of families that's hereditary, that they're carrying in their genes that are causing them to be much more vulnerable to the development of melanoma than other people around them."

DW: And it goes beyond that inheriting fair skin and light hair?
SL: "It does. In fact, there's some people in those families that really you wouldn't suspect would necessarily be so vulnerable, and yet they do get a melanoma. So you asked me about this p16 gene you've been hearing about. It's really important that everybody understand that every single person in the world has a p16 gene. Everybody has one. The problem with p16 is that in patients who have a mutation in p16—in fact, p16 is very, very important for the normal functioning of every cell in your body, and so if you have a mutation in p16, then that makes you vulnerable to getting a melanoma. And again, the data's not completely clear about exactly why that's true, but we think it has something to do with the fact that the melanocytes that are growing for some reason aren't growing under quite as good of control when they have a mutation in that p16 gene as they should be, and that tends to, for some reason, predispose them to turning into a skin cancer."

DW: That clears up a lot of questions that I had about the p16 gene. There was a little bit about the—is it the p22 chromosome?
SL: "That's a very exciting new breakthrough, so I love the fact that you're asking about this, because it means you've done a little bit of homework."

DW: I try to [do my homework].
SL: "Yeah, no, that's great! Now, what Danielle's referring to is, there's always, in cancer genetics and in research, one of the things, one of the holy grails is to try to find new genes that if there's a mutation in it, it makes you more susceptible to melanoma, because it would be sort of an equivalent to finding another p16 gene, a different gene that causes the same properties, right, an increased risk for melanoma. And there is a group of investigators in Arizona and around the world who have come together who are interested in hereditary melanoma, melanoma that runs in families, who have done a research project, a very extensive research project, looking for new genes. When you start to look for new genes, the way that you do it is you first have to locate on what chromosome that gene might be, because you can't just go directly for one out of thirty thousand genes; you can sequence all of them. So what you do is, you try to find the location of the gene, and then look within that region to see if you can find the exact gene that's causing the problem. And these investigators published a paper that showed that they think that they found a region in chromosome 1, and then p means the short arm, and 22 is the location along the short arm of that chromosome 1.So that's all that means. And it's very exciting news; it means that they're on a gene hunt, basically. Now they've got a region, now they can start to look more carefully for which gene it is in that region that's causing the problem."

DW: This is fascinating information! Dr. Leachman, what tools are being used in the research of these different chromosomes that we were just talking about?
SL: "Well, there are all kinds of different approaches. There's pretty much a straightforward linkage analysis, which was partially developed here in Utah that's a pretty powerful way to do it, and there are multiple other more advanced technologies that are on their way to being developed: using snips and things like that that are little polymorphisms, little small changes in the genes to try to more carefully dissect out the exact region. So there's a variety of techniques that are being used all over the world to try to locate genes. In fact, several different methods are being applied to the new gene hunt that they're doing on 1p22. So it's not just one particular method that's being used."

DW: I know that over at Huntsman Cancer Institute, you're continually putting together this database on different kindreds to better understand the familial links to melanoma. What if someone doesn't know their family history, they aren't sure who in their family has melanoma, if any, but they have a lot of moles, particularly atypical moles, and they want to have an assessment done on their personal risk for getting melanoma? What kind of steps could they take to identify that?

SL: "Yeah, that's a really good question. Not everybody does know their family history, and in fact, I want to make sure that I say before we finish the show that the people who have familial melanoma, the ones that we were talking about where there's three or more members of the family that have melanoma, are really fairly rare, probably between 5 and 10% of all melanomas, so it's not a very large percentage of the melanomas that we see. So that means that the majority of people, probably 90 to 95%, that have melanoma have a sporadic melanoma.

"But we do know that there are other risk factors that you can see within an individual, besides having to look at the family history. There are other clues that you can see in a single individual that would give you a hint that they're at higher risk for melanoma. Those things include some of the things that you just said, exactly what you were talking about—an increased number of moles; somebody who's a really moley person, is at higher risk for getting a melanoma than a person who doesn't have a lot of moles. Similarly, the kind of moles that you make; if you make large or very atypical moles, then those people are at higher risk than people who don't make those kind of moles, whether they have a lot of moles or whether they don't.

"And then there's some other risk factors that I think I'd like to go over, if you don't mind, because I think that's something for your listeners to really be aware of, that anybody who has very fair skin, who doesn't really tan very well and burns very easily is at risk, and that's regardless of whether they've had a lot of sunburns. If you add sunburns on top of that, that puts you at even higher risk. Another thing that you inherit from your parents but you can't control; things like red hair, very light blue eyes, freckles, all of those things also contribute to an increased risk for melanoma. And of course, if you've had melanoma already, that puts you at much higher risk for getting another melanoma.

"So all of those are risk factors that you can assess in a single individual, and you look at the whole person, based on the risk factors that they have, and you sort of give them an idea about how much higher risk they are. But I really think that basically anyone who is at increased risk for melanoma, even if they just have one risk factor, they probably deserve to have an evaluation by a dermatologist, by a good dermatologist who's interested in doing a thorough, total-body skin exam, looking at all of the skin on their body to make sure that they don't see anything dangerous. That dermatologist, based on their collection of the information about their risk factors, can then advise them on an individual basis what they think they need to do.

"Certainly a self skin exam once a month is a really powerful, powerful thing that every individual can do. I think most people are really familiar with a self breast exam—women have been told that for a long time—but people who have a higher risk for skin cancer, they need to do that exact same thing with a self skin exam once a month. And then, a routine exam with the dermatologist and being aware of what you're looking for. What do they mean that you need to look for something "new or changing"? And they have the A, B, C, D's that I'm sure you've probably already reviewed on this program, which is just the atypicality—what makes it look atypical. I sort of like to go with the idea that if you look at your mole and there's a spot in it that's growing differently than the rest, that's a sign that there might be something wrong. That would represent those cells that had turned on you."

DW: That's a perfect lead-in to the next question I was going to ask you, which is: Typically, melanomas (well, I should say, typically, skin cancers) are found on sun-exposed parts of the body—allegedly. But melanomas can appear anywhere there is skin. But what are the most common places for melanoma to occur for men and women? The next part of that was, how can we identify them? You talked a little bit about that already; if you would expound on that. Where the most common are places for melanoma to occur on both men and women, and are men or women at higher risk than the other?

SL: "Right, right, those are all excellent questions. The most common place on men is on the upper back, to have a melanoma, and the most common place for women is on the lower leg. But both of those areas are relatively common in both sexes, when you're talking about where the melanomas occur. Men tend you have a higher risk for getting a melanoma than women; it's not clear why. We don't know why. We don't know if it has something to do with the hormonal differences between men and women, or if it has to do more with the sun exposure differences between men and women, the fact that maybe men sunburn more than women sometimes. So we don't have really strong data to tell us for sure what the reason for the differences in the sexes is.

"Women, on the other hand, are the ones who identify those melanomas better than the men. So in themselves and in their family members, the women are the ones who are watching out a little bit better, and I would encourage all those men out there to get on the ball, and to start taking the lead from the women on this thing and start watching their wives a little bit more carefully too. It's hard for anybody to watch their back, or their scalp, or between their toes. So—get some help, you guys. Act as a team. That's what I'd like to encourage."

DW: Well said. I love that—work as a team. And you're right; women, for some reason—at least the ones I know—tend to notice those kinds of changes in the people that they love. I know that I do that. A lot of my friends do that. At any ray, I am curious about some research that I was doing earlier that was saying that melanoma is usually resistant to radiation and chemotherapy drugs that are designed to eliminate the cancer through cell death. How are the researchers at your lab studying this disease to better understand the molecular basis for that resistance?

SL: "Yeah, yeah! I want to brag a minute if I can. One of the researchers here at Huntsman Cancer Institute, a physician, another MD/PhD, his name is Doug Grossman, he works here at Huntsman Cancer Institute with me, and he's really on the forefront of trying to discover exactly why melanomas are so resistant. There is a property about cells that is called apatosis. It's basically a programmed cell death, where when the cell is damaged, or when it's not behaving properly, it's not growing properly, there are natural mechanisms inside of the cell to say, "hey, wait a minute, something's going wrong. We've got to self-destruct so that we don't turn into a cancer." Those mechanisms are exactly the ones that get triggered when you treat with radiation or when you treat with chemotherapy. In addition to being directly toxic, what they do is they trigger an apatosis. They trigger this self-destruction, because they damage the cells enough to where they say, "wait a minute, and I can't go on. I can't survive. I have to kill myself or else I'll be really abnormal." So one of the things that Dr. Grossman is really trying to discover is why that's true. And he has a lot of research; I would encourage everybody to go to the Huntsman website and take a look at his website, if they're interested in finding out more about that, because he really is an outstanding asset to the whole program here.

"Now, you asked why. We don't really know the answer to that yet. I wish I could tell you a little bit more. But they do tend to have this resistance to apatosis. Dr. Grossman studies a particular gene called survivin, where it looks like in melanoma cells, this gene is turned on, and as it's name implies, it causes it to survive in situations where it probably should self-destruct. So that may be one very important part of why melanoma cells don't respond properly to radiation or to chemotherapy."

DW: That is extremely interesting, Dr. Leachman. Back to its [melanoma] resistance to chemotherapy and radiation: when someone is diagnosed with a stage four melanoma—it's aggressive, it's metastasized, what kinds of treatments are provided for individuals like that, considering what we just talked about?

SL: "Well, you've hit exactly on the problem—that currently; there really are not any very good treatments for advanced melanoma. That's why it's so important to do those self skin exams, and do the preventative things, because once you've got an advanced melanoma, that's spread to other parts of the body, the survival rate is really low—it's probably about 10 to 15% only of people who survive, despite all chemotherapeutic efforts, all radiation therapy efforts, no matter what you do, it's very, very difficult to survive melanoma when it's advanced like that. Now there are a lot of trials underway, and some of those trials look to be promising, but they're clinical trials. Sometimes at that stage in development, one of the most powerful things that a melanoma patient can do, and most hopeful, is try something new. I encourage patients who are interested in participating in clinical trials to really consider doing that. We're constantly striving for progress against this disease, and in order to achieve progress, we do need help from the patients who are suffering from the condition."

DW: Oh, definitely. Backtracking just a little bit, if someone were to get diagnosed with melanoma, what's the process? In other words, what are the different types of biopsies that are performed, the kinds of questions they should ask if they wanted to get a second opinion just to be sure that that diagnosis was accurate, and—you get a pathology report, of course, and how to make sense of what that pathology report says, kind of deciphering the medical terminology—things like that?

SL: "Well, I think that is sort of a loaded question, because I don't think there's any one path toward the answers in getting that education and that information; I think there are multiple paths. Certainly one of the things that we have here that would be available to anybody who is seeking answers such as those is a wonderful Learning Center here at Huntsman Cancer Institute, and in Utah, we are happy to try to help direct patients to getting those answers, wherever they might lie, so if there was a question about a path report, and the terminology, if it was something that the educators down in the learning center can answer, they can answer it directly; if not, they're always, constantly seeking the advise of the appropriate person to provide that advice. So if it's about a pathology report, they might as a pathologist. If it's about a clinical issue, they might call me or one of our colleagues here. If it's about a clinical trial, like we were talking about a couple of minutes ago, trying to get into one of those. So it just depends on exactly what the issues and the questions are. I guess my single piece of advice would be that you need to get in touch with someone who really can communicate with *you* about what your questions are; somebody who's willing to take the time and make the effort to do whatever it takes to get those answers."

DW: That's excellent advice. I don't want to keep you too long, because I know you've just rushed from clinic right onto our show, and I'm sure that you have a full day still ahead of you. Before we let you return back to the Huntsman Cancer Institute, I'm so curious—I know that you were recently in the Netherlands, giving a conference. Would you be willing to share a little bit about that with us?
SL: "Sure, sure! It was a very exciting meeting. This is a meeting specifically dealing with melanoma genetics, and so the meeting was centered around discussions about the latest advances that have been made toward understanding the genetic basis of melanoma and why people who inherit mutations in p16, and why people who inherit presumed mutations in yet undiscovered genes, are at such risk. The really wonderful thing about that particular meeting is that you get a worldwide perspective. By bringing different people from all over the world, everybody comes from a different culture with a different perspective about how dangerous melanoma is, about what kinds of strategies need to be taken for melanoma, and about things even like how do you report back genetic test results about melanoma. And those are the kinds of things that we discussed, both formally, through didactic presentations that each group gives, but also informally, during dinner sessions and things like that. It was a very dynamic and exciting meeting, very productive."

DW: It sounds like it. Wow! Just before we wrap up our conversation with you, are there any points or issues that you would like to mention that we didn't ask you during the show that you want to make mention of now?
SL: "Well, I guess I would like to just keep coming back to one of the things that is the most near and dear to my heart, in terms of our program, which is the prevention, sort of the mission that we have about prevention of melanoma. I think that right now it's not that I don't support treatment and don't support all of the endeavors on diagnosis and all of that, but I think with what we're doing in my

clinic with the genetics, what we're really looking at is we're saying, 'okay, these people are at very high risk. How do we intervene to prevent them from ever having to go through a melanoma?' If we could prevent [skin cancer] then we wouldn't have to worry about treating it. And so I think that, especially in Utah, where there is such a really dramatic environmental risk factor that's associated with development of melanoma and other skin cancer, that prevention has the potential to cause the biggest impact on overall care for patients. That's very near and dear to my heart, and I hope that anybody who's interested in helping join us will get involved in any way that they feel appropriate."

DW: That's perfect that you said that, Dr. Leachman, because I remember the very first presentation that you gave for an event that the Cancer Crusaders sponsored was at Salt Lake Community College over a year ago, and the title of your presentation was *An Ounce of Prevention*. I what remember most is something you said at the end of your presentation. It was 'an ounce of prevention is worth a pound of treatment,' which sounds cliché but is so very true and what can we do to potentially not just decrease someone's likelihood of getting melanoma but perhaps spare them. [...] Thank you, Dr. Leachman, for taking time to share your knowledge. We appreciate the partnership we have with you, and wish you continued success with all of your endeavors over at Huntsman.
SL: "Oh, thank you very much and you guys keep up the good work as well. We like to see the young people out there starting with the grassroots, creating a real movement."

How sunscreen works and how to maximize sunscreen efficacy
Featuring Dr. Elma Baron of Case Western University
(Interview conducted by Danielle M. White and Kathleen E. Moncrieff on September 12, 2005)

DW: Dr. Baron, we would like to talk about the fact that there are so many myths and misconceptions floating around in the media about sunscreen and how to properly use it, does it really help us, is it really necessary, things like that. For starters, before we get into the nitty-gritty about sunscreen usage and the ingredients, would you be willing to address some of those common fallacies, and kind of clear those up for our listeners?
EB: "Yeah, sure. Well, first of all, let me say that sunscreen use is really one of the most effective strategies that we are advocating in order to prevent sun damage. By sun damage, I mean skin cancer plus the other effects of sun exposure, such as

the acute sunburn or the redness that you get. You can talk about the other things such as photoaging or wrinkling, but it's really the most extensively studied agent that we have so far in the market that can help prevent the damage caused by ultraviolet light exposure.

"There are many errors right now in terms of how sunscreens are viewed and how sunscreens are used, actually. And the latter is probably more important. For starters, we know that one, the amount that the general public is applying is less than the ideal amount that could really afford protection against UV light. You probably know that you need about a shot glass or about 30 ml of a sunscreen preparation to cover the entire sun-exposed areas of the body in order for it to be effective. Yet, surveys have shown that in general, people are applying probably just half of that amount. Half of that amount will not really give you the SPF protection that the bottle indicates. So that's one thing—that the public is probably applying way less than what is recommended.

"Another thing is that we are often skipping areas in the body. I know it sounds strange, but there are some areas of the body that are often missed in applying sunscreen. In some of the studies that have been done, the areas that have been missed were the ears, the mid-upper back (and I can imagine that, because it's kind of hard to reach that area). Interestingly, in melanoma, the most fatal of all skin cancers, the highest incidence is on the back. So we have to be wary of that and make sure that we are applying evenly on the back as well. Or have someone apply for you if you can't reach it!"

DW: I usually get someone to help me there, too! I can't reach parts of my back, especially since I broke it!

EB: "Yeah! And there are also certain portions on the legs that are often missed, and I don't know why; you know, it's pretty accessible. So there definitely are areas of the body sometimes skipped when using sunscreen. And of course, if they're not protected, you will get the sunburn, you will get the sun damage.

"And then the other thing is about the issue of application. Most people think that once they've applied, they're fine, and that's not true. Reapplication is probably one of the most important factors that we want to stress, because it has been shown also in studies that, among beach-goers for instance, that very few, probably 25%, of people on a regular day on the beach are aware of the fact that they have to reapply after two hours. Most people would apply right before or at the start of their sun exposure, and then they don't care, no matter how long they stay under the sun."

KM: And then they wonder why they get fried.

EB: "Right! Interestingly. There was this survey, actually, that was done, I think it was in Galveston, Texas, and I think about 70% of people who claimed that they had applied sunscreens were wondering why they got sunburnt. When everything was analyzed, it turned out that those who did not get sunburn were those who reapplied after two hours or so. So reapplication is definitely important. So I would rank those as the top three errors in the way that we use sunscreens at the moment."

DW: Well said, Dr. Baron, thank you. And, just to reemphasize what you said, Dr. Baron, Kathleen and I usually work mostly with college-aged students, here at The Cancer Crusaders Organization, who really aren't all that interested in learning about skin cancer as it is anyway because they don't want to face the fact that they are mortal, and they're more concerned about passing their midterms than they are about using sunscreen, but when I tell them, 'an easy way to remember is the 30-20-2 rule; You put it on about 30 minutes before you're ready to go outside; reapply it within the first 20 minutes of being outside, and then reapply it at least every two hours.' Then, the students lament, saying 'I have to remember to put sunscreen on at least 30 minutes before going outside?' I tell them that it takes you at least that long to get ready in the morning, put the sunscreen on when you're getting ready in the morning. It takes me at least 30 minutes to get ready in the morning.

KM: Me too.

EB: It takes guys three minutes to get ready in the morning.

DW: I suppose that's true. Another issue, too, is that not every sunscreen is created equal.

KM: We were actually just talking about that, about the ingredients you need to look for, and there are so many different sunscreens out there, so—do you have any tips on how to find the best sunscreen for particular skin types, and to fit with people's particular lifestyles?

EB: "Sure. But first of all, let me emphasize that all skin types should be using sunscreen. Because although we say that the light-skinned people are the most susceptible to skin cancer, skin cancer can also be found in other skin types, so it's not exclusively just the light-skinned individuals that have to be using sun protection. When choosing a sunscreen, right now we have the SPF—one of the factors we look at is the SPF value. And you have a range in the market. I've seen SPFs as high as 45, 60, and so on and so forth. As far as the American Academy of Dermatology is concerned, our recommendation is an SPF of at least 15, as a standard. So that's one thing, to look at the SPF value. Make sure your sunscreen is at least SPF 15.

"However, SPF only tells you how much the sunscreen protects against sunburn. And you know what, if you wish to call it "sunburn protection factor," you may as well call it that, because that's exactly how it is measured. The end point is really how much redness you get, or how much sunburn do you get with the sunscreen on. So the higher the SPF, the more protection against sunburn. But you have to keep in mind that sunburn is just one of the many things that UV light causes. And even before sunburn sets in, we know that there are already changes in the cellular, molecular level that's going on. So it's not enough to gauge the level of sun protection just via the SPF. So another thing that you should definitely be looking at is what we call the spectrum of coverage. In most products this would be labeled as broad-spectrum, or wide-spectrum. And that indicates whether the sunscreen has particular protection against UVA. You know that ultraviolet light from the sun is composed of UVA, UVB and UVC. UVC we don't worry about because it's the job of the ozone layer to filter that out. So we worry about UVA and UVB. Now the SPF label takes care of that UVB, because most of the sunburn effects of the sun is due to UVB. So if you have an SPF of 15 or higher, then you know that more or less, for regular daily exposure, you are well protected against UVB. The SPF value has nothing to do with how well the sunscreen protects against UVA."

DW: Isn't UVA the more dangerous?
EB: "It is the more penetrating, because of the longer wavelength. If the wavelength is longer, it reaches deeper into the skin. So yes, it is more penetrating. You know, years ago, we thought that UVA was actually okay, because it didn't cause sunburns. It caused tanning—and you know, a lot of people want that."

DW: Because it stimulates your melanocytes.
EB: "Right, exactly. More recent studies have shown that UVA contributes to skin cancer. UVA contributes to melanoma. So UVA is not better at all. It's just as damaging as UVB. So how do we know if a sunscreen has protection against UVA? Unfortunately, we do not have a standardized method of labeling UVA

protection, to the degree that the average consumer will say, 'oh, this is good' or 'oh, this is bad UVA protection.' It's not like the SPF, that we have numbers to go with that. For UVA, you really have to look at the ingredients of the sunscreen, because there are specific ingredients that cover UVA or that protects against UVA. These include, if I could mention ... actually, I'm trying to figure out how to make this really easy for people to remember"

DW: Actually, most of our listeners are college educated. They aren't experts, of course, but they are college educated, so—go for it.
EB: "I usually narrow it down to two ingredients, because these are the two ingredients that have protection against the longest UVA wavelengths. We set certain cut-offs for that, and there are a lot of studies that support this, but if you have to remember three names, two ingredients that have sufficient protection against UVA, that would be titanium dioxide, and the second would be zinc oxide. Now, the other sunscreen ingredients would have protection against maybe the shorter wavelengths of UVA, and of course the wavelengths of UVB. But if you want to narrow it down to which of the ingredients offer sufficient protection against long-wave UVA, which would be titanium dioxide, and zinc oxide."

DW: That's right. Literally. Thank you for clearing that up. This is very fascinating. We're actually going to go to a quick commercial break, and then we're going to come back and talk to you about finding—you gave us a great base—finding the right sunscreen that is right for your particular skin type, for your lifestyle, and for your budget.

KM: Dr. Baron, if you would give us some tips on how to find the best sunscreens for your skin type, budget, and lifestyle?
EB: "For skin type, there are really no definite guidelines. We go by the dictum that all skin types have to use sunscreen, and we base our selection of sunscreens on one, the SPF, and two, the broad-spectrum protection, whether it has the ingredients that would afford UVA protection. I know the sunscreens come in different vehicles, also. You know, there are lotions, creams, gels, sprays, sticks; in general, the stickier it is, like creams and ointments, would last longer than the water-based formulations. So it depends on your lifestyle, but regardless of what you use, even if you're using the stickiest product, these are not waterproof. So if you're sweating, like when you're running, exercising, and especially when you're swimming, you have to remember to reapply often."

DW: Is there really such a thing as a sweat-proof, waterproof? Isn't that misleading?

EB: "Yeah, it's misleading. But they should be labeled as "water-resistant," which means that it's not waterproof, but there's a certain amount of time of immersion in water or sweat wherein they still maintain their SPF activity. So there are some products that would maintain their activity after eighty minutes of water immersion. There are some that would only maintain their SPF activity within forty minutes of water immersion. So in general I say you have to reapply every one and a half hours or so if you are in a wet situation—if you're swimming or you're sweating."

DW: I go swimming all the time, so that's good to know. Also, for the kids under eighteen; isn't it recommended that the parents put that on their kids every hour?

EB:" I think we base that on, you know, usually they're hyperactive, and running a lot, they can rub against things, and so that may affect the substantivity of the sunscreen on their skin. But I'm glad you mentioned kids, because we would like to emphasize that sun protection definitely has to begin in childhood. As early as they start going out and playing under the sun, they should be using adequate sun protection. We know that by age eighteen, you probably have received the majority of the UV exposure that you would receive in your lifetime. So you have to start early."

DW: In fact, if I remember correctly, the American Academy of Dermatology was saying that approximately eighty percent of your lifetime sun damage.

EB: "That's correct."

DW: Speaking of that, that leads perfectly into the next question that Kathleen and I had for you. What is your professional advice, from your own experiences as an educator and as a researcher, how we can increase sunscreen usage, particularly among children and establishing that lifelong habit of proper sunscreen usage, proper sun safety from day one?

EB: "We have to talk to the parents. We have to convince the parents more. Behavioral studies have shown time and again that parents who are conscious of sun protection will also have children who are conscious of sun protection. Another means is probably the school system, and there are ongoing studies on that, on how effective is the incorporation of sun protection education, like in elementary schools? It would be too late if we did that in high school, we want to do it early on. So yeah, we're constantly searching for venues to make this available and understandable and applicable to children."

DW. Actually, when we talk to college students, we get that question get often: 'why are you talking to college students? They've already sustained most of their damage.' Yet, my take on that is that young adults are going to be parents, if they aren't already, and they're entering the workforce, so they can, hopefully, with that knowledge, take that with them when they're going into parenthood, the workplace, and then perpetuate that culture of sun safety.
EB: "I agree."

DW: Go back, if you don't mind, Dr. Baron, back to the discussion on sunscreen ingredients; what about the sunscreens out there on the market right now that aren't broad spectrum, that don't employ ample amounts of proven effective agents such as the zinc oxide? Is there any sort of FDA standard on that? Who regulates and monitors to make sure that our sunscreens are properly protecting our skin?
EB: "Well, sunscreens are classified as over-the-counter drugs, and so yes, they are FDA monitored, to an extent. And yes, we have sunscreens out there that are not optimal sunscreens. They will afford some protection, but they will not afford total protection, not at all. They may be able to prevent some of the acute damages of sun exposure, such as the acute sunburn, but then in the long run, you do not derive any benefit from that, or you do not derive as much benefit as you would derive from an optimal sunscreen."

KM: We often get people saying things to us about they've heard that you need to be out in the sun to make vitamin D and that if you use sunscreen, you won't have enough vitamin D and that'll cause problems. Could you clarify for us?
EB: "Oh, I would love to clarify that because it's not an excuse to be exposing yourself in the sun just to derive vitamin D. First of all, about sunscreens and vitamin D: there are no studies that have ever confirmed that sunscreen caused a significant decrease in our vitamin D levels, or that sunscreens caused an enhancement of the diseases that are associated with lower levels of vitamin D, such as osteoporosis. No, sunscreens have not been shown to do that, to adversely affect our vitamin D system. Do not worry that you will be vitamin D depleted if you are using sunscreens.

"Now, how much sun exposure do you need to generate vitamin D? The answer to that is: very little. The daily exposure that you get, you know, maybe from just your driving and walking from your car in the parking lot to your office and back, with your face, your neck, and your hands and arms exposed, is sufficient to generate vitamin D. They're coming up with better guidelines on how much vitamin D we need, and I agree with that; we really have to establish how much vitamin D we really need to prevent disease, but regardless, I don't think you should use UV light, which is already a proven carcinogen, to generate vitamin D. There are other sources of vitamin D that are non-carcinogenic, so why should you resort to something that causes skin cancer to get vitamin D? I tell my children to drink milk, to try to obtain it from the diet instead of going to a tanning salon or going outside and getting a sunburn."

DW: That's true. Americans fortify most of their grocery products with vitamin D as it is anyway.

KM: That's right, breakfast cereal, dairy products, etc.

DW: If I remember right, our friend Natalie was at the last meeting for the National Coalition for Sun Safety and she was saying that she learned that having a bowl of cereal every day even gives you an adequate amount of vitamin D to sustain your bone and your calcium. And yes, thank you for pointing out that UV rays are proven, known carcinogens, which means cancer-causing, in all organisms, not just humans, and for pointing out too that incidental sun exposure by being in your car, or going to and from the mailbox, whatever, is sufficient too. UV rays can penetrate through the windows.

EB: "Oh, definitely."

DW: Speaking of UV rays, has any research been done or any data collected that illustrates the relationship between UV rays and the rising skin cancer incidence, even the skin cancer mortality? I'm sure there is.
EB: "Well, you know, the data stems from a lot of different studies, both in the laboratory just looking at what UV rays can do to skin cells, to actual epidemiologic studies, and seeing whether sun exposure truly affects the incidence of skin cancer. And the answer to all of that is yes. UV rays directly contribute to skin cancer growth. And we're talking not just melanoma, but of course the more common skin cancers are actually the non-melanoma skin cancers, which are the basal cell carcinoma and squamous cell carcinoma. So whether non-melanoma or melanoma skin cancers, UV has been proven as a main environmental causative

agent. Not to say that genetics do not play a role; we all know that there are certain races, certain backgrounds that are prone to skin cancer, but if you take all that together and just focus on what is the environmental agent that definitely contributes to skin cancer growth, it is without question. That's UV light."

DW: Re-emphasizing the sunscreen issue, because that's our main subject for today—Because we work so much with the young adult population, we, of course get the relentless laments: 'but it gets in my eyes,' or 'it makes me break out; I get acne.' As a mother and as a doctor, having both perspectives, what is your advice on what we can do to kind of dispel their laments and re-emphasize that it is important to use sunscreen?

EB: "Right. Well, talking about the eyes, it is true that sunscreen ingredients can irritate the eyes. So our advice is to avoid direct application on the eye. But as far as breaking out, getting reactions, you know if you do controlled studies on these, the chance of getting that is actually minimal. For example, for allergic reactions, some people say 'but I do get allergic reactions to sunscreen,' I would say try a different sunscreen.

"Because there are so many other UV filters or sunscreen ingredients available, it doesn't mean that if you react to one you will react to the others. It's really a matter of finding the right formulation for you, and unfortunately there's no clear-cut formula that'll tell me when I see a patient, 'oh, you will definitely not react to this.' I cannot say that. It's just a matter of trying it out, and trying the other options if this one does not work well for you, if you get a breakout or get a different reaction to this one. But what I can say is that right now there are so many formulations that are very compatible with most skin types, whether you're oily-skinned, or dry-skinned. It almost should not be a problem anymore. And you know that makeup is also incorporated with sunscreen ingredients. I hear some people tell me, 'so I'll put on the sunscreen and then I'll put on my makeup, and then my face will be three inches thick,' but it doesn't have to be that way. There are already foundations and powders and all that that have a certain degree of SPF in them. And moisturizers, too, have some SPF in them, so it's not like you have to be putting five products on all at once. And you can tailor it to whatever your skin type is and whatever you think fits your skin."

DW. One last question for you, because we know you a busy woman, Dr. Baron. There was a statement issued by the American Academy of Dermatology that quotes you about in the future of sunscreens. It said: 'increased understanding of sunscreen protection against immune suppression could result in more optimal sunscreens for people who are more prone to UV damage and skin cancer.' Would you be willing, Dr. Baron, to expound a little bit on that? I thought that was intriguing.

EB: "Well, one of the harmful effects of ultraviolet light that we don't really appreciate so much is immune suppression. UV light suppresses immune functions for skin. And we believe that contributes also, at least partially, to the formation of skin cancer. If your skin's immune system is down, you lose that surveillance mechanism that tells you early on, 'oops, there are bad cells that are starting to grow.' So when we're evaluating sunscreens, one of the aspects that we're looking at also is its capacity to prevent sun-induced immune suppression. And there are certain assays that are devoted to that. I believe that that's definitely an important thing to look at, because immune suppression is definitely contributory to skin cancer. We're not there yet; we're not at a point where we can say, 'oh, this sunscreen protects the immune system by this much.' Again, it's not like an SPF, that I can provide a number for every formulation, but we're working toward that. And just this month, September, we published a paper in the Journal of Investigative Dermatology—actually, a consensus paper, it was worked on by us and experts from around the world, on developing assays as to how we can measure the immune protection that's afforded by a sunscreen preparations. That's really new—hot off the press!"

DW: And, we get to be one of the firsts to know about it! How wonderful!
EB: "Yeah, that's some work that was done by us at Case Western and a photo-protection group in the UK, a group in France, a group in I believe Austria, and a group in Australia, specifically on immune protection. This is a very novel thing. We're starting to introduce that; we want people to understand that also, that aside from sunburn, your skin's immune system is also getting suppressed. And you know what's more interesting, is, we've found out that this immune suppression can actually take place even before the sunburn sets in to the skin. So again, the sunburn is not your endpoint. You cannot say that, 'oh, I'm fine, I did not get a sunburn,' because there are other things happening that you do not see."

Student Essay

Compare/Contrast Essay
of the Tanning Industry

By Maile Wilson
"Only Skin Deep?" Peer Educator's Training & Certification Program
Final Essay
September 1, 2006

In the ancient times, cultures throughout the world would worship the sun. They even went as far as to name the sun, Apollo, which referred to the Sun God that brings life giving heat and light to the earth. These people also thought of the Sun as a perfect sphere of celestial fire created by the Gods.

Over hundreds of years there have been many culture changes involving the way society viewed the sun. These numerous changes defined different wealth classes as well as helped define who you were as a person.

Skin color became one of the ways to separate the working class from more wealthy classes, and separated the master from his servants. Darker skin indicated a life of outdoor labor, while pale skin belonged to the leisure lifestyle of the upper class. The paler ones skin the higher the class, and men and women went to great and sometimes unhealthy lengths to be pale.

Due to how important these men and women thought it was to be light some would even use lead paints and chalks to help whiten their faces. Not known to the people at the time, these treatments could and did lead to slow deaths caused by lead poisoning. Another way that woman would attempt to make themselves look whiter came about during the reign of Queen Elizabeth. Instead of painting their whole faces white, now they would just paint blue lines on their forehead in order to make their skin appear translucent, which in turn made it appear paler. As well as that, anytime they would go outside they would either carry a sun umbrella or wear a mask in order to hide their face.

It wasn't until the twentieth century that society once again changed its view of the sun. Starting during this time period people throughout the world began accepting the bronzed skin look. This change has been blamed on two French celebrities.

In the nineteen twenties fashion designer Coco Chanel started to alter the way women viewed and wore clothing. She got rid of the once confining styles for more relaxed and comfortable trends that women all over the world were starting to admire. Due to this people everywhere were looking to her for fashion advice and to see what she would come up with next. While she was on a trip from Paris to Cannes she once again had the opportunity to change another fashion trend. It is said that this one was probably unintentional; she got a suntan from all the time that was spent out doors. Due to this she turned it into a new fashion style.

This new-bronzed look really got the attention of both men and women throughout the world, because as fashion trends were changing so were peoples lifestyles. It was becoming acceptable for women to come out of the house and enjoy the outdoors. Society would now view women as still being sexy and feminine while hiking, playing tennis, going on picnics and doing various other activities such as these. Fashionable women everywhere threw away years of tradition to be tanned.

Clothing began to cover less because these women wanted to show off their newly tanned skin. Shoes with stocking became unheard of, and bathing suits, that had once covered a women's leg with bloomers, now bared the legs, and swimming became acceptable and popular. Beaches across the world which had once been a spot that no one would dream of going with out being overly covered were now filled with hundreds of women sunbathing.

The period of the sun tanning had arrived. Being tan, which was once the sign of the working class, was now the symbol of a lifestyle full of wealth and leisure. Having tan skin during the winter month's meant you had enough money and status to afford a vacation to an exotic, warm climate, or snow sports in winter villas.

By the nineteen seventies, an entire generation had baked their bodies in the sun, totally oblivious to the fact that the suntans they had obtained in their youth would develop into skin cancers ten to twenty years later. Since this time there have been hundreds of thousands of hours of research done in order to find links between the UV rays from the sun and the development of skin cancer.

Over the years skin cancer has become one of the most common types of cancer, resulting in more than half of all new cancer cases reported. This is due to society's view that a person must have a bronzed look in order to be healthy. Sometime around the nineteen thirties the chance of an American developing Melanoma, the deadliest form of skin cancer, was one in fifteen hundred whereas nowadays it has risen to one in thirty-four. More frightening than this is that one in five Americans will develop some form of skin cancer during their life. Even though these statistics are extremely high in the United States they are even worse in counties like Australia. Greg Hunt, Federal Parliamentary Secretary for the Environment who has the responsibility for the Bureau of Meteorology, states that "around 380,000 Australians, almost two per cent of the population, are diagnosed with some form of skin cancer each year. This means that approximately, fourteen hundred Australians die of skin cancer annually. Also every year, doctors remove around 720,000 lesions from the skins of Australians because they are suspected skin cancers."

This dramatic increase is due to a number of alarming factors. Some of these to be discussed are as follows; people not understanding the importance of covering up and applying sunscreen while outdoors, ozone depletion which causes a stronger correlation between being out doors and becoming sunburned, also the increasingly popularity of tanning beds.

Most people feel that it is only children that need to use sunscreen, and with that, they only need to apply it while at a beach, lake, outdoor pool, or other planned outdoor activities. This is not true! Everyone needs to use sunscreen! Studies have shown that especially in Australia, skin damage can happen within as little as fifteen minutes of sun exposure. Due to this, one in five Australians gets sunburned on typical summer weekends. The sun puts out two types of harmful rays, UVA and UVB. These rays are the very strongest between the hours of 10:00 a.m. and 4:00 p.m. It would best if a person could avoid going outside during that period, but since that is unrealistic everyone just needs to be cautious and apply proper sunscreen and clothing.

When choosing an appropriate sun block it is very important that a person gets one that blocks both UVA and UVB rays, which is referred to as "broad-spectrum" sunscreen. Also it needs to have a minimum of a sun protection factor (SPF) fifteen for the best protection. If a person is going to be outside spending a lot of time in the sun it is very important that they reapply their sunscreen every two hours, putting about one ounce on each application. It might be necessary to apply sunscreen more often than that depending on the amount of time spent swimming or sweating.

Since these precautions all tie together, it is important to know why there is a higher risk factor for developing skin cancer today than there was a hundred years ago. It has been said by NASA, "The use of "external environmental factors" refers to ozone depletion and the subsequent increase in UV irradiation and exposure, which has circumstantially contributed to at least 90-percent of skin carcinomas." Besides just having NASA's findings, The Environmental Protection Agency has released information saying that, "As of September 2003, the earth's ozone has a hole equivalent to the size of North America that will potentially result in an estimated 40-million skin cancer incidents in 2005." Another group of scientists belonging to the National Research Council stated, "That just a 10-percent global loss of ozone results in a minimum 26-percent increase in skin cancer incidence meaning that a 1-percent decrease in ozone layer triples the increase in UV-B radiation."

This problem of ozone depletion is even worse in Australia than it is in the United States. This is because Australia is located beneath an extremely large hole in the ozone layer. Due to this, the country as a whole has the highest skin cancer rate in the world, but they are taking action in order to help prevent future people from getting this horrible cancer.

Australia's government in order to help combat the countries extremely high risk for getting skin cancer has started issuing a thing called The Sun Smart UV Alert. Greg Hunt, Federal Parliamentary Secretary for the Environment who has responsibility for the Bureau of Meteorology, said this: "The Australian system was based in part on a similar system in Germany. The intention of the alert system was to educate Australians that ultraviolet radiation, not temperature, was what caused skin cancer." This is reported and printed daily in the newspapers, and broadcast during all of the weather forecasts throughout the whole country. The alerts purpose is to raise the public awareness of the risk they are in every time they leave the house due to over exposure to these harmful UV ray. Kylie Strong, a member of the Cancer Council Australia's National Skin Cancer Committee, states that, "The UV index levels tend to be higher during the middle of the day but people are getting sun burnt outside of the hours 10-3." The index encourages people to take proper safety precaution while outdoors, even if it is only for a few minutes. The UV index has a variety of levels going from less than two all the way up to eleven plus, it gives categories anywhere from low to extreme which are all paired up with a color and certain safety precautions. UV levels are determined by a number of factors being; latitude, cloud cover, time of year and time of day. Due to this, the people of Australia have had a hard time understanding that the UV index can and usually does change every day and the government is trying as hard as they can to get this point across. It is totally dependant on which month and season the country is in. Any time the UV index reaches a three or above skin damage most commonly sunburn can occur, this increases the likely hood of obtaining skin cancer. The UV index is a measure of the maximum daily level of ultraviolet radiation. Each day the reports will change and give the exact information for that day. An example of this is listed below:

UV-Index Level	Exposure Category	Precautions
2 or less	Low	You can safely stay outdoors with minimal protection.
3 to 5	Moderate	Wear a hat, sunscreen, sunglasses, seek shady areas.
6 to 7	High	Wear a hat, sunscreen, sunglasses, seek shady areas. Stay indoors between 10am and 2pm (11-3 daylight saving time).
8 to 10	Very High	Stay indoors as much as possible, otherwise use all precautions above.
11 or higher	Extreme	Same as previous category above.

It has been proven time and time again that ultraviolet radiation causes skin cancer. Neither UVA nor UVB rays are good for a person, so why is the indoor tanning industry becoming more popular? The tanning trade publications report that, "this as a five billion dollar a year industry in the United States, and estimates about, twenty eight million Americans are tanning indoors annually at about twenty five thousand tanning salons around the country." In the years two thousand two, the federal Government's National Toxicology Program listed, "broad-spectrum ultraviolet radiation, whether from sunlight or sun lamps, as a known cause of both melanoma and the less lethal forms of skin cancer in humans."

After all the research that has been done against tanning beds, the American Academy of Dermatology has labeled them as, "the health-peril equivalent of cigarettes. All have urged prohibiting their use by minors. If adults want to make the decision to use tanning beds, fine," said Dr. James M. Spencer, clinical professor of dermatology at the Mt. Sinai School of Medicine, proposing regulations to bar minors in tanning salons. "But we don't sell cigarettes to minors, and indoor tanning is similar—we know it will cause cancer. Not maybe. Not might. It's going to cause cancer. No one under 18 should be allowed to use those things." With all of this evidence states have begun trying to pass tanning regulations for minors.

Since the year two thousand three, nineteen states have successfully been able to have laws passed that restrict children under the ages of eighteen to be able to tan. Although some states have tried none of them have been successful at banning all teens from using tanning beds.

There are also new laws in New York and New Jersey, which ban all children under fourteen from using tanning beds; these are among the toughest in the nation. Only California's law is as strict. In Massachusetts, Texas, Tennessee, Illinois, Florida and Louisiana, for example, children under fourteen are allowed to visit tanning salons if they are accompanied by a parent. In Michigan, the statute only suggests parental consent.

One of the main reasons that the government and dermatologist across the country want tanning banned is because a number of studies indicates links between melanoma and getting a sun burn early in life. That is what tanning beds are doing to these young people; they are burning in order to create a tan look. This is the same skin that twenty to thirty years later will be leather looking, wrinkled and at a possible risk for getting skin cancer. An analogy that I once heard went something like this; your skin is your body's largest organ. You wouldn't consider putting any of your bodies other organs, such as your lungs, brain, liver or kidney out to fry, would you, so why do it to your skin? Not very many people think of skins importance when they are lying in a tanning bed. They are just thinking of the quick-bronzed look that will perfectly compliment their new prom dress, swimsuit or everyday look. If these young girls only understood that a tan is not a symbol of good health, which is something that I have heard so many time, it is really a sign of too many UV rays, in fact enough of them to damage the skin. Due to this common misconception, Melanoma, the most fatal form of skin cancer, is the most common cancer in young women aged twenty-five to twenty-nine, according to recent dermatological studies. One of the main reasons for this is because; seventy percent of all the people that go to tanning beds annually are Caucasian women between the ages of sixteen and forty-nine.

Part of the reason that the strict laws that prohibit teens from tanning can't pass is because of groups like the Indoor Tanning Association, which represents several thousand tanning parlor owners and equipment distributors nationally. They hired a lobbying firm out of Washington and claim, that nearly thirty million people safely use tanning facilities each year in the United States. The executive director, John Overstreet said, "Dermatologists have been trying to link indoor tanning to skin cancer for twenty years, and there is no proof. Melanoma takes years to develop," he said. "So for them to say that we are causing an

increase in melanoma among young people—well, it's the opposite of the truth."
Legislator, Patrick J. Moroney of Pearl River, was quoted during a public hearing
saying the following regarding tanning regulations, "So a teenager can have an
abortion but not get a tan without her parent's consent?"

"The tanning industry will say there is no study that says if you go to tanning
salons you will get cancer, and they're right; we're all exposed to sun from the day
we're born," said Robin Ashinoff, the Director of Dermatologic Mohs and Laser
Surgery at Hackensack University Medical Center in New Jersey. Also, Tanning
Trends magazine, a trade publication, writes: "Moderate tanning has never been
linked scientifically to skin cancer. In fact, by helping people tan with a reduced
incidence of sunburn, indoor tanning may reduce your risk of ever contracting
skin cancer." Besides these statements, during the last year the tanning industry
has taken a stand. They claim that indoor tanning is not only harmless, that it is
actually quite healthy.

Indeed, quite the reverse is true: by increasing exposure to UV rays, the risk of
skin cancer is increased no matter what the tanning industry says. In the year
eighteen ninety four the first association between sunlight and skin cancer was
discovered. P. G. Unna of Berlin published a report discussing it. Since that time
there have been a number of clinical and laboratory studies done to support this
claim. That, UV radiation seems to be the cause of all three common skin cancers—basal cell carcinoma, squamous cell carcinoma, and melanoma. The UV
rays are thought to increase skin cancers by three mechanisms: "First, ultraviolet
light directly damages DNA leading to mutations; second, it produces activated
oxygen molecules that in turn damage DNA and other cellular structures; and
third, it leads to a localized immunosuppressant, thus blocking the body's natural
anti-cancer defenses."

Tanning beds have not been proven directly to cause skin cancer but there is
enough evidence to prove a strong correlation between the two. Why would anyone want to take a chance and put him or herself in such high risk? If the bronzed
look is so important there are hundreds of self-tanning products on the market
that give off the same appearance without the damage. Each only takes a few
hours to start working and with no chance of the burned flesh sting.

To those that are passionate about skin cancer education, the possibility that
using tanning beds can increase the risk of skin cancer is enough reason to make
laws that will protect children. Hopefully through getting out the message to
more people about the dangers of both UVA and UVB rays the occurrences of
skin cancer will lower and fewer individuals will have to go through hearing a
doctor give the bad news. It only takes a few minutes to cover up and put on

proper amounts of sunscreen in order to help lower ones risk. Just follow two simple sayings: One quoted by The Cancer Crusaders Organization is: "Slip, Slap, Slop! Slip on a long-sleeved shirt. Slap on a wide brimmed hat. Slop on SPF 15 sunscreen everyday." The other from the Utah Cancer Action Network, it goes as follows, "It's as easy as your ABC's; A= Avoid the sun in the middle of the day; B-Block the sun by applying sunscreen; C= Continuously take sun safety precautions."

(Reprinted with permission by The Cancer Crusaders Organization)

Bibliography

ABCs of Skin Cancer. New York: American Academy of Dermatology, 2002.

"All about skin cancer." The Cancer Council Australia. December 2004. The Cancer Council Australia. 1 Aug 2006
<http://www.cancer.org.au/content.cfm?randid=960742

Australian Government. Australian Radiation Protection and Nuclear Safety Agency. Australian UV-Index. 2006.
<http://www.arpansa.gov.au/uvindex/daily/ausuvindex.htm>

Davie Sean. "Frequently Asked Questions About Indoor Tanning." Email to Pacific Sun Co.

Edelman, Hope. Motherless Daughters. First. Dell Publishing, 1994.

Familial Melanoma Research. Utah: Huntsman Cancer Institute, 2002.

Fischetti, Mary. "Tan or Burn." Scientific American. 1 Jul. 2001.
<http:www.sciam.com/article.cfm?articleID=000A376-D620-1C6F-849809EC588EF21>.

Goask, Alice. "Seasonal Depression." E-mail to author. 11. Nov. 2002.

Guidance Notes for the Protection of Workers from Solar Ultraviolet Radiation.

New Zealand: Occupational Safety and Health Services, January 2000.

Aric-Romine Merry. Health Effects of Ozone Depletion: Skin Cancer. September l2003.

Health Effects of UV-B Light. NASA. 1993.
<http://www.nas.nasa.gov/About/Education/Ozone/radiation.html>.

Human Health Effects. National Research Council. March 1979. Ciesen Thematic Guides 1986 http://www.ciesen.org/docs/001-534/001-534.html.

Is the Sun Good or Bad? Deschenes S. October 1999. The Federation of Canadian Naturists 20 Oct. 2003.

Journal of the American Academy of Dermatology, 1990, 22(3): 449-452; Kaidbey, K.H.

Karrow, Julia. "Skin So Fixed." Scientific American. 1 Mar. 2001. <http://www. sciam.com/article.cfm?articleID=FB4-8944-1C70-84A9809EC588EF21>.

McCarthy, Will. "Thin! Tan! Hotter Than Hell!" Wired. 1 Jun. 2002 1 <http://www.wired.com/archive/10/16/melanotan.html>.

Mobley, Barbara. "Extension Launches Skin Cancer Initiative. Newsline 334. (2003): 15 pars. 20 May. 2003 <http://www.aces.edu/dept/extcomm/newspaper/may20a03.html>.

Only Skin Deep? Utah: The Cancer Crusaders Organization, 2003.

"Ozone levels return to unhealthy status." Houston Chronicle Online 11 Sept 2003. <http//www.chron.com/cs/CDA/ssistory.mpl/topstory/2088661>.

Prevention of Skin Cancer by Reducing Exposure to UB Light through Mass Media Interventions. Sarayia Mona. September 2003. Centers for Disease Control and Prevention 11 Sept. 2002 <http://www.thecommunityguide.org/cancer>.

Reece, Gabrielle. Big Girl in the Middle. First. Crown Publishers, Inc.,1997.

Reifler, Ellen J. "Why I Hate Pink Ribbons." Herizons: July 1997: 25-26.

"Safe Tanning." totaltravel.com. 2006. totaltravel.com. 1 Aug 2. 006 http://www.totaltravel.com.au/library/traveller/medical/safetanning

Scottery, John. "How Does Sunscreen Protect Skin?" Scientific American. 1 Oct. 2003.   <http://www.sciam.com/askexpert_question.cfm?articleID=00062AD1-59E8-1C72-9EB78>.

Scotto, J.A. W. Kopf, and F. Urbach. 1974. "Non-melanoma Skin Cancer among Caucasians in Four Areas of the United States." Cancer. 34: 1 May. 1974: 1333-1338.

Seasonal Affective Disorder. American Academy of Family Physicians. September 2000. American Academy of Family Physicians 2 Feb. 2002.

Skin Cancer. New York: National Cancer Institute, 2002.

Skin Cancer Awareness Foundation and Environmental Protection Agency. 29 Oct. 2003 <http://skincaf.org/partnetships.html>.

Skin Cancer and Outside Work. Workcover Authority Labor Council. January 2002. Unionsafe 9 May. 2003. <http://unionsafe.labor.net.au/hazards.html>.

Skin Cancer Prevention among Construction Workers. June 1995. International Union against Cancer & Pilot Study in Netherlands 20 Mar. 1996. <http://www.uicc.org/others/ecp/ecp2908.htm>.

Skin Cancer Scares to Prominent Americans Bring Message of Sun Safety to Light. The American Board of Plastic Surgery. March 2002. American Society of Plastic Surgeons 27 Mar. 2002. <http://www.plasticsurgery.org/news_room/press_releases/Skin-Cancer-1. Scares-to-Prominent>.

"SunSmart UV Alert." SunSmart. July 10, 2006. The Cancer Council Victoria. 25 Jul. 2006 <http://www.sunsmart.com.au/uvalert>.

"Sun Tanning." Cool Nurse. 2006. Cool Nurse. 21 Aug, 2006. <http://www.coolnurse.com/tanning.htm>.

"SOLARIA." SOLARIA Cologne. 2005. Koelnmesse. 21 Aug, 2006 <http://www.solariacologne.com/>.

"The Case Against Indoor Tanning." The Skin Cancer Foundation. 21 Aug, 2006 <http://www.skincancer.org/artificial/>.

Thomson, Hilary. Skin Cancer Patients Know the Risks but Fail to Act. August 2003. University of British Columbia Public Affairs 7 Aug. 2003. <http://www.publicaffairs.ubcca/ubreports/200303aug97/skincancer.html>.

UV alerts to help combat skin cancer." Sydney Morning Herald December 4, 2005. <http://www.smh.com.au/news/National/UV-alerts-to-help-combat-skin-cancer/2005/12/04/1133631137640.html>

Vitello, Paul. Skin Cancer Is Up; Tanning Industry a Target." <u>New York Times</u> <u>August 14, 2006, New York Region</u>

White, Danielle. "<u>Only Skin Deep?</u>"® <u>Peer Educator's Training & Certification</u> <u>Program</u>. First. Lulu Press, Inc., 2006.

Whitmore, Elizabeth." Tanning Salon Exposure and Molecular Alterations." <u>Journal of the American Academy of Dermatology.</u> May 2001. <http:www.fcn.ca/sun.html.>

<u>Why You Should Know About Melanoma</u>. Georgia: American Cancer Society, 2002.

978-0-595-43273-8
0-595-43273-5

Printed in the United States
73393LV00004B/1-15